Praise for *The Heart-Centred Doctor*

Dr. Olivia Ong MD uses her own lived experience to share 12 ingredients of a *recipe for wellness and fulfillment for the modern physician*. Things they don't teach in medical school like self-compassion, gratitude, mindfulness and more. She illustrates each one with stories from her own life as a pain physician and her personal journey back from a spinal cord injury that forced her to learn to walk all over again. Her stories and these ingredients will help the physician reader put more heart and soul back into your life and your practice.

Dike Drummond MD, USA, CEO, TheHappyMD.com

This is a moving and powerful personal account of a physician who has navigated the detours of life with grace, strength and dignity. Dr Ong has allowed herself to be deeply vulnerable about her life journey so as to provide practical hope and encouragement for others. These are the kinds of things they don't teach us in Medical School. Her life story is a testament to the truth and principles written in this book. I am grateful for Dr Ong's courage in sharing her life with us. I believe many will find inspiration in these pages.

Dr Eric Levi, ENT Surgeon, VIC, Australia

This book provides all health professionals who are interested in the area of wellness within oneself with a contemporary understanding of how the brain, mind and body connect. What triggers in one, is registered in another. It is a heartfelt guide that explores the recurrent theme confronting doctors in the ever demanding and changing sphere in medicine. Olivia has harnessed the wisdom she has developed from her own personal experience of burn out and shows us how to look after the emotional wellbeing of the physician. I encourage anyone who struggles with their work life balance and its effect on them emotionally to read this book.

Dr Clayton H Thomas, Rehabilitation and Pain Physician, VIC, Australia

In The Heart-Centred Doctor, the author provides a raw, honest and courageous account of one doctor's struggle through her own personal circumstances in the face of an unrelenting system that encourages putting everything else before self-care. Through self-compassion Dr Ong shares her story of overcoming tremendous adversity and shares her insights with both doctors within the system and the wider readership. Part self-help book, part autobiography, Dr Ong leads the reader on her journey, her struggles and what enabled her to achieve a better and happier work-life balance. I wish I had read this book as a junior doctor, to know some of the pitfalls that come with career progression, the difficulties of the system and recognition of burnout and most importantly, learning a framework and tools in order to prevent this.

Dr Noam Winter, Anaesthetist and Pain Physician, VIC, Australia

Dr Olivia Ong described in this book her journey and struggles as a female doctor and how she learnt and grew from her unfortunate experience of spinal cord injury. She showed much authenticity and passion in helping other doctors. I enjoy reading this book and appreciate the "secret ingredient" she learnt and shared. Many doctors, in particular, female doctors, who struggle with professional, personal and family demands will resonate with her experience. This book provides many practical tips that many doctors would find handy to help handle many challenges as doctors, to grow, and to become a more resilient, happier, and fulfilled person. I strongly recommend this book.

Dr Aston Wan, Pain Physician, VIC, Australia

This is such a unique heart-warming book. It combines information giving on "how to be a heart-centered doctor" and the inspiring story of Dr Olivia Ong's personal journey of surviving a spinal cord injury and still live life to her full potential. It is so unique it combines Dr Ong's inspiring journey surviving spinal cord injury and educating the concept of self-compassion to medical professionals who people assume doctors know it all but in fact we are the most vulnerable group.

Dr Angela Chia, Anaesthetist
and Pain Physician, VIC, Australia

As a friend and colleague, I was honoured when Dr Olivia Ong invited me to read and review her book. Dr Ong has captured both the light and the dark of medicine, uniquely, from both the perspective of patient and practitioner. Her narrative leaves the reader with much food for thought for both the care giver and basic human within all of us about the importance of attending to the needs of self, labelling thoughts and feelings that many of us have but perhaps, push through to our own detriment. Congratulations and thank you Dr Ong, for sharing your inspiring and empowering experience, and tools for growth.

Dr Bethany White, Anaesthetist
and Pain Physician, VIC, Australia

The Heart-Centred Doctor

Dr Olivia Ong

First Published by the Power Writers Publishing Group in 2021.

2nd Edition published by the Power Writers Publishing Group in 2022

Copyright © Olivia Ong 2021.

A catalogue record for this book is available from the National Library of Australia

NATIONAL LIBRARY OF AUSTRALIA

ISBN 978-0-6452588-2-0 (pbk)
ISBN 978-0-6452588-3-7 (ebk)

Typesetting and design by
Publicious Book Publishing
www.publicious.com.au

Disclaimer
Any opinions expressed in this work are exclusively those of the author and are not necessarily the views held or endorsed by others quoted throughout. All of the information, exercises and concepts contained within the publication are intended for general information only. The author does not take any responsibility for any choices that any individual or organisation may make with this information in the business, personal, financial, familial or other areas of life. If any individual or organisation does wish to implement the ideas discussed herein, it is recommended that they obtain their own independent advice specific to their circumstances.
The content of this book is general in nature, provides no individual clinical advice, and in no way replaces a medical consultation. Readers are advised to contact their own doctor or other health professional in relation to any clinical concerns they may have.

This book is available in print, and ebook formats.

Dedication

To my husband John and my children,
Joseph and Jacqueline - You are my inspiration.

To my Daddy and Mummy
Thank you for encouraging me to pursue my dreams

To my brothers Andrew and William
Thank you for always supporting me and having my back

Contents

Foreword

This book is nourishment for your soul.

To say that this is timely is an understatement. It seems like everyone is focused on the COVID situation at the moment, but this effectively masks a much darker scenario that no one is talking about. It is the dire situation that medical practitioners worldwide are working within.

Dr. Olivia Ong knows firsthand what the price to be paid is, if something isn't done about this. The victim of burnout herself, and the survivor of serious accident that left her in a wheelchair, Dr. Ong is uniquely positioned to be able to shed light on what is going so terribly wrong inside hospitals from both sides of the fence. As a pain physician, she knows exactly what it is like to care for patients in a seriously dysfunctional system.

Above all else, this is a book about hope written by a big-hearted doctor who punches well above her weight. Her diminutive frame doesn't prepare the unwary for the power of her message. This is a woman on a mission to make the world a better place - one doctor at a time.

This book is about arming doctors and others within the medical profession with a number of simple but effective tools to keep themselves well. The key tool here is self-compassion.

Helping you to find your way back to your soul is what this book is all about. With any luck, putting the oxygen mask on yourself first will become second nature to you, and you won't have to go through what Dr. Ong and countless others have gone through in the way of physical and emotional breakdown.

I think you're going to be inspired by this book. And I hope that you take the messages within it to heart.

— Jack Canfield, Co-author of the *Chicken Soup for the Soul*® series and *The Success Principles*™: *How to Get from Where You Are to Where You Want to Be.*

Prologue: The Awakening

It was a sunny autumn day in April 2020 when the reality of the first wave of the COVID-19 pandemic was starting to hit home in Australia. I'd just eaten breakfast with my family when the news reported on an emergency physician from New York State who had jumped off the roof of the hospital she was working in. This really shocked me. My heart sunk for the poor doctor and her loved ones as I reflected on the fact that this could have been me.

Twelve months later, I'm putting the finishing touches on this book. Needless to say, Covid hasn't gone away. It has affected us in so many ways. Some of us have lost loved ones. Others have lost jobs or businesses. The politicians are talking about their roadmaps to economic recovery. But it strikes me that very little is being said about emotional recovery.

My name is Dr Olivia Ong. I am a pain physician working in public and private practice in Melbourne, Australia.

As a pain physician, I'm in the position of witnessing my patients not only having to deal with physical pain but also emotional pain. I can say, from firsthand experience, that the mental health impacts of Covid have been massive. In fact, it is the emotional impacts that worry me the most. Social isolation, loss of loved ones and livelihoods and increased levels of uncertainly in general, have led to higher levels of anxiety and depression. The flow on from that is a spike in the consumption of opioid medications. This is a problem because these are highly addictive substances and people can get into a lot of trouble with them if they're not careful.

My particular focus is on the wellbeing of doctors. The question of who is caring for the carers is top of mind for me. The truth of it is that physician burnout was at epidemic proportions before the COVID-19 pandemic. According to research presented at the 2018 American Psychiatric Association Meeting, 400 physicians die by suicide each year in the US. This is double the rate of the general population. In fact, doctors have the highest suicide rate of any profession in the US – including combat veterans.

One thing the pandemic has done is expose the cracks in the healthcare systems around the world. From inadequate testing and personal protective equipment (PPE) to overcrowded emergency departments, frontline staff are putting their lives at risk to care for highly infectious patients. Regardless of the fact that the odds are stacked against them, medical professionals are responding to the crisis with characteristic selflessness, resilience and compassion. It strikes me as profoundly unfair, not to mention strategically unwise, for the people who are being relied on so much to be left to suffer in silence – to the point where jumping off a building looks like the best option.

For many physicians, COVID-19 was the straw that broke the camel's back. Being isolated physically from family and friends, and overwhelmed by the surge of sickness and death they face on a daily basis, means that depression, anxiety, post-traumatic stress disorder and secondary trauma are reaching levels that have never been seen before.

I had several conversations with my brother, Andrew, during the second wave of the pandemic in May last year. Andrew is a gastroenterologist in Singapore. He was deployed to the frontline and socially isolated from his family. He told me about the stress and anxiety he felt around the PPE process in particular. The reality for him was that one wrong move in putting on or taking off his PPE could result in him contracting Covid. I was really worried about him after this conversation. The long hours wearing PPE, with equally long gaps between meal and comfort breaks, had definitely taken a toll on him. I could only imagine the emotional pain he was experiencing because of the extended separation from his wife and two young kids.

I also had a conversation with one of my friends who is an anaesthetist in Australia. She told me about the stress she was under as part of the intubation team looking after patients who were severely ill with Covid and in respiratory distress. My friend is the mother of a 4-year-old girl and was constantly worried about getting Covid and either passing it on to her daughter, or (worst case scenario) leaving her daughter without a mother. On one level, I know that kind of fear, but on the level of day-to-day lived experience, I can only wonder about what resources my friend needs to just get through each day.

I had another conversation with one of my patients who I'd been looking after for about two years. Among other things, he lost his job during the pandemic and the state of his mental health forced him to reach out for help. He was particularly distressed about not being able to say goodbye to his father who was in palliative care during the pandemic. The day he received the call advising him that his father had passed away, he was actually with us in the clinic. He dropped to his knees and just sobbed and sobbed. His emotional pain was so palpable we were all vicariously impacted with a sense of loss and grief.

For my own part, I fell hard during the pandemic. I was at my worst in July 2020 when we went through a stage 4 lockdown in Melbourne. Melbourne is the part of Australia that has fared worse for one reason or other. However, comparatively speaking, the death rate from Covid in Australia is fantastically low, with less than 1000 deaths being recorded up to the end of May 2021. I had not long given birth to my daughter, Jacqueline, when we went into lockdown. My hormones were all over the place and I was recovering from a caesarean section when I found myself socially isolated at home with a newborn baby and my 5-year-old son, Joseph. Before long, I found myself spiralling down into a vortex of despair. To get through this, I had to dig deep and access resources I didn't even know I had.

The silver lining of the pandemic, from my point of view, is that it brought virtual mentors to me. I signed up for a life-changing, online intensive course held by the Center for Mindful Self-Compassion. My virtual mentor, Kristen Neff, taught me the practices of self-compassion that enabled me to deal with difficult emotions and put an end to the kind of negative self-talk that was particularly prevalent when I was at my lowest ebb. The most significant result of putting what I learnt into practice was that I started to love myself more. That happened as I was implementing a number of simple but profound internal and external self-care strategies that helped me to be a much more mindful, self-compassionate and patient mum to my children.

Self-compassion entails acknowledging that we are suffering, that we are all in it together and that we need to love and be kind to ourselves before we can really do the same for others. For the first time in my life, I found a place of peace and power within myself through self-compassion. I believe that creating a ripple effect from self-compassion is the best way forward for us as a collective. Essentially, that is what this book is all about.

Medicine is a calling for most doctors – but is it worth dying for? I don't think so. The way I see it, we all have a role to play in stemming the tide of physician burnout and suicide. The time has come to reaffirm the humanity of doctors and acknowledge their value to society. Medical culture and the healthcare system both need to change – that's the bottom line.

Doctors must first acknowledge, and then heal, their pain and suffering with self-compassion. They have to do this for their own sake first and then for the sake of their patients and communities.

I have learnt a number of heart-based tools that helped me find my way back home to my heart and I'm sharing these with you in this book. My mission is to arm doctors and other medical professionals with the tools they need to tap into the heart-centredness of medicine.

As a nod to my love of food, I decided to structure this book around the idea that each of the principles or tools are an ingredient in the dish of life. Self-compassion is the hero ingredient. The other ingredients are Faith, Intuition, Mindfulness, Freedom, Vulnerability, Gratitude, Energy, Alignment, Boldness, Love and Belonging.

I look forward to taking you on the journey to the centre of your heart through self-compassion.

And if you're anything like I used to be, you might be feeling incredibly time poor and wondering how you're going to find the time to even read this book. If that's the case, you might like to jump ahead to Chapter Twelve right now. I've written that chapter to not only wrap up what's gone before it, but to stand on its own in terms of giving you the core strategies from the leadership program I developed called The Five Keys to Freedom. If you start there because you're stressed out and time poor, you'll be able to use the strategies I share to claw some of your time and energy back and invest that in reading the rest of the book, and a whole lot more.

Wishing you all the best.

Olivia Ong

The Heart-Centred Doctor

———————————

Secret Ingredient One: Faith
Choosing faith over fear

My mother, Agnes, grew up in Surabaya in Indonesia. My father, Daniel, was from Jakarta in Indonesia. My parents met in 1977 through a mutual friend. It was love at first sight and they got married the following year. I was the 'honeymoon' baby. I was born in Singapore where we lived for two years before moving back to Indonesia. I was three when my brother Andrew was born, and six when my youngest brother, William, joined us.

I started school in Jakarta when I was seven. I learnt all of my subjects in Indonesian, so I had to repeat a year when we moved back to Singapore for my father to pursue business opportunities. I was on the back foot and remember feeling embarrassed because I couldn't speak English when I started school in Singapore. Eventually, I picked it up and managed to do relatively well with my grades – so much so that I sat the entrance exam and successfully got into one of the top primary schools in Singapore. I started my studies at Nanyang Primary School in 1989. I really enjoyed reading books when I was a kid. Writing and telling stories brought me joy because I got to use my imagination and creativity. My world was all about unicorns and rainbows back then because, like many little girls at the time, I was literally in love with *My Little Pony*.

I was brought up in a Christian environment and, from the age of eight, went to Sunday School with William and Andrew. I enjoyed reading the stories in the Bible because I felt like I was really able to connect with the characters.

We travelled a lot as a family when I was growing up. My parents often took my brothers and I all over the country by car as they travelled from place to place, meeting people about their skincare business. It brought me so much joy to see the beauty of nature as we drove past rice fields, mountains and villages during our road trips in Indonesia. We also travelled internationally – to places like Los Angeles, Hawaii, Paris and London. I really loved learning about the culture and history of other countries.

After I completed the Primary School Leaving Examination at Nanyang Primary School, I was accepted into the Raffles Girls' School. This was the top girls' high school in Singapore. The year I crossed the threshold from primary school to high school was 1993. That's the same year that Whitney Houston released her Grammy Award-winning song, *I will always love you*. If you're anything like me, that tune will now be like a mind worm that you'll have playing inside your head for a while. Apologies for that.

I loved my high school years. My principal and teachers taught me to be an empowered and confident young female leader. Our school motto was 'Daughters of a Better Age.' I remember feeling idealistic and inspired, and imagined being able to impact the world with my vision and purpose one day. Academically, I excelled in geography, history and biology. I guess this makes sense because I loved travelling and learning about the history of the places I visited. I'd also always had a fascination with the human body.

Another great outcome of my time at the Raffles Girls' School is that I became part of a wonderful bunch of like-minded friends.

Like teenage girls all over the world, we spent our spare time together watching movies, reading comic books and listening to pop songs by boy-bands like Take That, Boyzone and Backstreet Boys. One of the other things about this part of my education is that I was surrounded by perfectionists and over-achievers. Most of my classmates wanted to be either lawyers or doctors. For my part, from as far back as I can remember, I have always wanted to be a doctor. Unlike others I know, my parents didn't force me to do medicine. They've always genuinely wanted me to pursue my heart's desire. I smile as I share the fact that, in some part, my passion for medicine was fuelled by my favourite TV show at the time, *ER*. Those were the good old days when George Clooney was the star of the show.

After I completed my O-Level examinations in Singapore in 1996, I was accepted into Singapore's top junior college. I spent two years at Raffles Junior College preparing for my A-Level examinations. This was around the time I started to be aware of the opposite sex. I was painfully shy around boys. The effect of my shyness was compounded by the fact that I was relatively overweight. This made me feel super self-conscious. So I kept to myself and focused on my studies. This suited me fine because I was determined to excel in my A -Level examinations so I could get accepted into medicine. I also volunteered in community centres and old folks homes. I wanted to give something back and I found the volunteer work very fulfilling. It was also wonderful to gain experience working with people with dementia and intellectual disabilities.

I was accepted to study medicine at The University of Melbourne in Australia after completing my A-Level exams. I was really excited by the idea of the independence I would have in Australia without my immediate family hanging around. My extended family was in Melbourne, though, and I looked forward to spending some time with them. So, in 1999, when I was twenty, I moved to Australia to study medicine. I stayed with my extended family for a month before moving to my own apartment near the university.

The years at university were the best years of my life. I made so many great like-minded friends, many of whom were international students like me. As well as studying a lot, my life was filled with things like going to the gym with my friends, having supper in Chinatown and potluck dinners on special occasions. I will be forever grateful to my parents for supporting me during my years at medical school. Those years gave me a solid grounding and a real sense of purpose.

I was getting ready to head to Singapore for my elective early in 2003 when it was cancelled due to the SARS pandemic. There are definite parallels between SARS, which was the first pandemic of the 21st century, and Covid. Of course, the impact has been quite different. SARS stands for Severe Acute Respiratory Syndrome. The outbreak in 2003 apparently started in Foshan in Guangdong, China. From there, it spread throughout China and then worldwide, as far as Canada. The outbreak officially ended on the 5th of July 2003 when the World Health Organization declared that SARS had been eliminated. By the time the infection was brought under control, there were 238 cases in Singapore, thirty-three of whom died. Along with Singapore, more than twenty other countries reported SARS cases.

Owing to the situation with SARS, I wound up doing my elective in neurosurgery at a tertiary hospital trauma centre in Melbourne. I was a fifth-year medical student at this stage and was very interested in pursuing a career in neurosurgery.

I graduated from The University of Melbourne as a doctor in 2004, when I was twenty-five years old. I remember the day of my graduation as if it were only yesterday. My youngest brother, William, and my parents were sitting in the audience. My parents travelled all the way from Singapore to attend and when the Dean of the Medical School called my name, it was with a genuine sense of pride and gratitude that I walked up to the stage and took my Bachelor of Medicine and Surgery and Bachelor of Medical Science certificates in my hand.

I started my internship in a regional hospital in Victoria in 2005. It was great to experience the country lifestyle for the twelve months of my internship. I really enjoyed my rotations through the areas of Internal Medicine, Colorectal Surgery, Upper Gastrointestinal Surgery and Emergency Medicine. I also enjoyed the close-knit medical community I was part of, as well as the community within the church at Hobsons Bay that my friend, Cathy, introduced me to. This was where I met my husband, John. Ours was not a case of love at first sight. We became friends first and our beautiful relationship slowly blossomed out of friendship and into marriage. Among other things, John was incredibly supportive of me throughout my internship.

I moved back to Melbourne after completing my internship and, in 2006, took up the role of Hospital Medical Officer (HMO) in a tertiary hospital. I worked as a surgical HMO for two terms in the area of vascular surgery. My bosses were friendly and approachable and so was my registrar, Dr James. I wasn't in a position to join the dots at the time but looking back on it now, it's clear I was witnessing Dr James being burnt out from the long hours he spent in vascular surgery. In many ways, it was a clarion call as I watched Dr James change from a kind and compassionate doctor to a very jaded and worn-out version of himself.

My years as HMO were a massive learning curve for me. I enjoyed the clinical experience and I really appreciated John stepping up and supporting me in every way during those years. John and I got married at the end of 2006. Our wedding day is another one of those days I remember as if it was only yesterday. I felt nervous and excited at the same time as I walked down the aisle with my father next to me and John waiting at the altar. It was as close to perfect as it could possibly have been with our dear family and friends celebrating our wedding day with us before we headed off to Thailand for our honeymoon.

My career took a new shape when the beautiful hubbub of the wedding was behind me. I got a chance to discover that I love the holistic and multidisciplinary approach of Rehabilitation Medicine when I spent a term as a Rehabilitation Medicine HMO in a subacute geriatrics and rehabilitation hospital early in 2007. Because of the experience I had there, I embarked on my Rehabilitation Medicine traineeship at the end of 2007. In the beginning, I really enjoyed learning about the various topics within the field of Rehabilitation Medicine and I loved working with the great trainees I connected with. Before too long, however, I felt myself losing heart. The reality of it was that I was working in a job that was highly analytical and I had to use my left brain for critical thinking almost exclusively. The long and the short of it is that I worked in a healthcare system that eventually left me feeling emotionally and physically burnt out. As a high achiever, I had a habit of beating myself up when I made even the smallest of mistakes. In fact, sometimes I even beat myself up in anticipation of making a mistake. Back then, the idea of self-compassion was an oxymoron. At best, it was perceived as a luxury and at worst, it was perceived as a sign of weakness. These days, I see self-compassion as a non-negotiable priority in my life.

You might have been wondering what the things I've been sharing with you here have got to do with faith, which is, after all, the overarching theme of this chapter. Here's the thing – what I know

now, with hindsight on my side, is that things would have been very different for me if I'd had faith in my intuition, rather than ignoring it and defaulting to logic as I was working with patients in the rehabilitation space. The bottom line is that my heart would never have veered so perilously close to being broken if I'd had faith in my intuition. You'll be hearing more about how this transformation came about soon.

Alas, I became jaded and disgruntled with medicine. I wound up in a state of despair because, somewhere along to track, I had disconnected from myself. It's no wonder I felt so miserable. The worst was yet to come because the last thing I expected was to suffer a traumatic spinal cord injury in 2008. This brought a whole new meaning and proximity to the idea of 'Physician, heal thyself.'

Secret Ingredient Two: Intuition
Choosing intuition over suppression

The 10th of September 2008 should have been a great day. I got out of my car and walked through the hospital carpark. It was the same path I took on most days. Out of the corner of my eye, I saw an old, worn out Toyota reversing out of the disabled parking spot. I didn't think much of it. Then, in the blink of an eye, I was thrown up in the air and landed with a hard thud on the ground. I opened my eyes and noticed excruciating pain in my lower back. It was one of those times when time seems to stand still. I remember thinking that I was lying in an awkward position and that the car I saw reversing must have hit me. Then I was struck by the idea that I was still alive and realised that God had protected me. I thanked Him profusely for saving my life.

I then put my rehabilitation registrar's hat on and did a head-to-toe inventory. My thinking was intact, so I knew I didn't have a traumatic head injury. I started moving my arms and concluded I was not a quadriplegic. Then I realised I wasn't able to feel my legs. That's when I panicked. I hoped against hope I was not a paraplegic but when I realised I was not able to move my legs, I knew I had a spinal cord injury. This is what the doctors call 'spinal shock' – where there is a loss of sensation, accompanied by motor paralysis, with complete loss or weakening of reflexes below the injury. When the injury is less severe, this phase usually only lasts for about a day with the neurons in various reflex arcs normally receiving what's called a basal level of excitatory stimulation from the brain. After a spinal cord injury like the one I had, though, these cells lose this input and the neurons involved become less responsive to stimulation.

Suddenly, a 'code blue' was called. I heard the words, "Code blue in the carpark. Code blue in the car park." A group of doctors rushed towards me. I recognised them. They were the rehabilitation doctors I was training with at the time. In that moment, I realised I was the code blue. The looks of concern on the faces of the people around me were impossible to miss. My intuition told me I was in for the long haul and that my life would never be the same again.

I asked Dr Robin, who was the senior rehab doctor on duty, whether I would be admitted to the main hospital where the car accident happened. Dr Robin avoided my gaze and told me in a soft tone that the hospital was on bypass because the Emergency Department was full. I would have to be transferred to another tertiary hospital. I looked at him angrily. I was really distressed by the fact the hospital was not prepared to take me. I was one of their employees for goodness sake!

The paramedics came swiftly and Dr Robin performed a clinical handover before they put me on the stretcher in the ambulance. The siren was on and I was on my way to one of Melbourne's major tertiary trauma hospitals. I was going there as a patient, not as a doctor. I remember feeling anxious when I realised no one had called my husband to let him know I was on my way to hospital because I had been involved in a car accident. I felt helpless and alone on the stretcher and wished someone were in the ambulance with me.

I waited for a long time in the hospital bay before John was finally able to come in and see me. Dr David, the orthopaedic doctor on duty, came and talked to me. He had a really compassionate manner. I can confirm there is no truth to the rumour that surgeons are a cold-hearted bunch with no compassion. I vowed that once all of this was over, I would emulate Dr David's approach and be a compassionate doctor like him.

Dr David organised for a CT scan of my lower back. It felt weird being in the scan machine for the first time. I noticed how cold the metal surface was as I was lying on the table and how cold the radiology room itself was. The scan was over in less than fifteen minutes and the porters whisked me back to the bay in the Emergency Department where John was waiting for me.

It felt like an eternity, but it was probably less than an hour before Dr David came back to fill me in on what the scan had shown. He looked sad when he arrived and my heart sank because, deep down, I knew things were not good. He informed me I had a burst L2 vertebrae with L1 and L2 dislocation in my lower lumbar spine. This can't be happening, I thought to myself. I was devastated. My life was ruined. John slumped in the chair looking absolutely devastated when he heard the news. We were both speechless as we looked at each other when Dr David told me I needed to have emergency spinal surgery that day. I signed the consent form with my hand shaking like a leaf.

My memory of being transported to the operating theatre is crystal clear. John was walking next to me as the stretcher glided along the corridor. I lost sight of John once I reached the operating theatre. In all my life, I have never been so scared and distraught at the same time. Thoughts were running through my mind, like: We have never been apart before. What if we end up being apart forever if I don't make it out of surgery alive?

I looked around the operating theatre with white cold fear coursing through my body and my mind. I closed my eyes and through the emotional pain I realised I was afraid I might die on the operating table. Dr David and his boss, Dr Susan, came in to speak to me. I noticed that Dr Susan was also very compassionate. She spoke to me about the details of the operation in a calm, gentle voice. I nodded and accepted my fate then and there. I remember the anaesthetist, Dr Sam, putting an intravenous line in and the next thing I knew, I was waking up in the recovery room. I was disorientated, but alive. John was sitting on a chair, looking completely exhausted. In fact, he was nodding on and off to sleep. In that moment, I realised I was really alive, and I thanked God for that.

The next two weeks were like hell on earth. I was experiencing acute pain in my lower back. The medication I was on made me drowsy and disorientated. Eventually, I had improved enough to be transferred to the rehabilitation hospital. I spent four months in the rehabilitation ward, learning how to live my life in a wheelchair. I learnt to use a slideboard to transfer myself from my bed to my wheelchair and back again. I noticed the sad faces around me. These were people who also had spinal cord injuries and were chained to a wheelchair like me. Like them, I had to learn bowel and bladder management from the specialist spinal nurses. I couldn't know what was going on for the others but I knew that while I might have been making steady progress on the rehabilitation front, the truth of it was that I had lost all my dignity. The experience of being a patient, rather than a doctor, was a traumatic one for me. I was receiving great medical care, but nothing was being done to account for the fact that I had lost all hope.

A couple of months into my inpatient rehabilitation stay, I was eating lunch in the dining room with a fellow patient, Gerry, who also had a spinal cord injury. We were talking about the movie dates with our partners that were scheduled to happen over the weekend. This was a trial run to see how ready we were to cope with going back into the community in our wheelchairs. Suddenly, Rick, another patient with spinal cord injury, came into the dining room. He had an air of excitement about him. I asked him what was going on and he started telling me about Project Walk – a rehabilitation centre in San Diego in the US that specifically helps people with spinal cord injuries to walk again. I got a bit excited myself when I heard about this. My intuition told me to pack my bags and head to Project Walk right then and there. However, overnight, I chose to ignore my intuition and just kept doing what I was being told to do by the spinal rehabilitation team at the hospital. I kept ignoring my intuition for a very long time, but I never gave up hope of walking again.

Let me turn the lens away from me and onto you for a moment. Have you ever heard your intuition telling you to follow your heart and pursue your dreams and then had 'logic' kick in, telling you that you aren't good enough or you aren't worthy or whatever? What did you do? Did you give up on your dreams?

Intuition, which is also known as gut feeling, is a vibe we get around something not being quite right. Experienced doctors often get a sense when a patient's story just doesn't add up. Intuition helps us make decisions in complex medical situations. Clinical evidence can only take us so far and, for anyone who is open to it, the heart and gut does the rest. Sadly, most doctors aren't open to it.

For my part, I'm incredibly grateful I was finally able to actually 'hear' my intuition, twelve months after I first learnt about Project Walk from Gerry. This was one of those defining moments, where your life is literally set on a path by choosing one option over another. It happened during the Christmas period in 2009, when I was lying on the bed with John in the supported accommodation we were renting while our house was being modified to suit my wheelchair. My intuition told me to pack my bags and leave for San Diego so I could check myself into the Project Walk Paralysis Recovery Center. Fortunately, my boss was totally understanding and supportive when I told him I was planning to go away for two years to focus on my rehabilitation. I was really touched when he gave me his blessings and told me to go ahead and strive for my dream to walk again.

I was full of hope as John and I packed our bags for the long-haul flight to San Diego via Los Angeles. There was no doubt in my mind about having made a heart-centred decision that was pointing me in the right direction. However, when we got to the airport the following day, I started feeling nervous. This was the first time I'd travelled internationally as a disabled person and a number of doubt-based thoughts went through my mind, like: what if the airline damages my wheelchair during the flight? I'm happy to report that everything went smoothly and my wheelchair arrived intact. In fact, this wheelchair still accompanies me on trips, both overseas and within Australia.

Secret Ingredient Three: Self-Compassion
Choosing self-compassion over self-judgement

What I've come to understand over time is that lots of people are 'paralysed' and living their life in an invisible wheelchair. They might be stuck in a job they hate, trapped in a loveless marriage, shackled in a number of unfulfilling relationships that are built on the principles of people-pleasing or any number of other situations that limit their ability to be truly happy and fulfilled.

I had been completely unaware that I was trapped in one of those invisible wheelchairs until I found myself having to rely on a real one. Paradoxically, it was the real wheelchair that showed me the way to free myself through self-compassion.

What is self-compassion?

Dr Kristin Neff is one of the leading experts in the science of self-compassion. She describes self-compassion by way of three key pillars.

Pillar one is mindfulness

The aim in this pillar is to acknowledge our pain and suffering and experience our emotions without suppressing them or exaggerating them. The thing to do is observe our emotions with mindful awareness, just as they are. This helps us to avoid getting swept up in unhelpful cycles of negative reactivity.

Pillar two is common humanity

Often, when we are suffering, we feel isolated. It is helpful to recognise that all humans suffer and that we are all imperfect. We can reframe the narrative and see that, rather than being isolated, we are participating in a shared human experience through suffering.

Pillar three is self-acceptance and self-kindness

The key is to be kind and gentle with ourselves when we face suffering, whether it manifests through failure, imperfection or through challenges outside our control. It is helpful to accept these things as a normal part of the human experience, rather than fighting against them and becoming angry, frustrated or self-judgemental.

You'll recall from Secret Ingredient One that I was working as a junior doctor in Melbourne prior to my spinal cord injury. In hindsight, it's easy to see I was mindlessly trapped in a stressful job that didn't satisfy me; yet I kept pushing through to please everyone, especially my bosses. This was the invisible wheelchair that keep me stuck and feeling overwhelmed all the time.

I paid minimal regard to my own needs as I carried out the responsibilities of my job on autopilot, which is the exact opposite of mindfulness. I was walking from ward to ward, looking at charts, hardly making eye contact with the patients, rushing off to organise chest X-rays in Radiology or whatever. At times, I was so busy I even gave myself a hard time for needing to use the bathroom. At one stage, I actually wished I could have an indwelling catheter inserted so I wouldn't need to pee. How insane is that?

For many years, I struggled to feel entitled to ask for help. I had been programmed to work as a lone ranger. One of the unofficial lessons we learnt in medical school was that seeking help meant being weak, not capable and not competent. This training sat very comfortably beside the fact that I was a perfectionist. Whenever I made a mistake, I would beat myself up with self-judgement on steroids. I probably ticked all the boxes for success on the outside but, on the inside, things looked quite different as I was going through extreme stress and burnout. It's an award-winning understatement to say I was not extending anywhere near enough compassion to myself to sustain the journey of being a doctor with my spirit and passion intact.

Experiencing the other side of the healthcare system was really good for me, although it didn't feel that way at the time, of course. The days I spent in the hospital were really difficult. Even though the evidence was stacked against me inasmuch as I couldn't move my legs at all for a few months after I had surgery, I was still not ready to accept I would never walk again. Meanwhile, I felt so vulnerable and helpless, with drips in my arms and a feeding tube up my nose, it took all the willpower I had at my disposal not to completely lose hope. I was engulfed by grief and loss. The questions that kept going through my mind were:

- Will I ever be able to walk again?
- Will I ever be a doctor?
- Will my husband leave me?
- Will I ever have kids?

The days following my discharge from hospital were the worst. It felt like the wheelchair was my enemy. I was terribly self-conscious. I felt every pair of eyes from every person I passed cut into my soul with a knife called pity. I also felt like I could sense relief in the people who tried to look away. It was as if they were relieved it wasn't them in the wheelchair. However, it wasn't other people who were the worst – in the ultimate act of self-hate, I blamed myself for the accident.

As you heard in the last chapter, learning about the Project Walk Paralysis Recovery Center in San Diego was a game-changer for me. The fact they had the latest, state-of-the-art technology for locomotion, such as exoskeletons and robotics, not to mention the expertise of the trainers, made the idea of travelling halfway around the world a no-brainer for me. I thought these were the things that would help me but not long after I arrived, I knew there was something much deeper going on at Project Walk. What I learnt when I was there between 2010 to 2012 is something much more powerful than how to use my legs again. I also learnt how to nurture myself through self-compassion.

The things I needed to be able to learn to walk again were the exact opposite of the things I drew on during my life as a junior doctor:

(1) Instead of being on autopilot, wishing I had an indwelling catheter so I wouldn't have to worry about going to the bathroom, I needed to be mindful of each and every muscle I used with every step I took.

(2) Instead of being a lone ranger and struggling to seek help, I needed to actively connect with fellow spinal cord injury survivors and be buoyed by the bond we had through our common experience of spinal cord injury.

(3) Instead of being a perfectionist and beating myself up for every mistake I made, most importantly, I needed to accept myself for who I was and rediscover the true meaning of self-worth.

Being self-compassionate boosted my spirits exponentially and I started doing amazing things in San Diego. I went hiking and kayaking with my trainers. Nothing could stop me once I reframed the situation I was in and focused on what I could do, rather than letting myself get bogged down with what I couldn't do.

Despite being in a wheelchair, I frequently went to Disneyland, going on all of the rides with the SoCal CityPASS I invested in. The SoCal CityPASS (otherwise known as the Southern California CityPASS) is a multi-attraction discount card. It also got us into SeaWorld in San Diego. There was something calming and mesmerising about watching the sea animals go about their business. I was incredibly touched, and even cried, when I watched Shamu the killer whale in the live shows. Shamu was just such a beautiful creature. This experience was a far cry from the shame and embarrassment I felt when I first ventured out in my wheelchair.

Another truly memorable experience I had involved a group of us going to Las Vegas for the 4th of July celebrations. Two of us were paraplegics. My husband, John, was the designated driver with responsibility for getting us there in the scorching heat of Nevada in summer. The car could have broken down at any moment due to the sweltering 100 °F temperature in the region, but we didn't care. This was an adventure we had been looking forward to for ages.

John and I became even more adventurous after our jaunt to Las Vegas, and we travelled to New York City not once, but twice. Words can't express how free I felt when I stood with my sticks (i.e. no wheelchair) at the top of the Empire State Building.

With great experiences like these peppering our time in the US, I never begrudged the five gruelling hours doing physical therapy every day from Monday to Friday. I knew I had taken a risk in going over to the US but after two agonising and wonderful years with Project Walk, I learnt to walk again. Physically, I had not totally recovered – there was still a long, long way to go – but emotionally, I had definitely turned the page. I was over the moon when I returned to Australia and, in August 2012, I went back to my job in Melbourne. I was happy, enthusiastic and ready to tackle new challenges when I walked back into my life as a doctor.

However, it didn't take long for the negativity of the system I left behind for a couple of years to start bearing down on me again. From where I was sitting, there seemed to be a lot of unconscious bias at play. My medical colleagues were sceptical about the results I'd achieved, and, for some reason, my competence seemed to be getting judged unfavourably by just about everybody. In fact, in the process of giving me a poor performance review, one of my previous bosses told me bluntly that my medical knowledge had deteriorated while I was away. Another previous boss made a huge deal about me having to use a wheelchair at work when I broke my leg in late January 2016. She insisted I speak to the Infectious Disease Team because she was worried about my wheelchair spreading germs from one room to another. There are many more examples I could be sharing with you here of the shoddy treatment I received when I went back to work at the hospital. Needless to say, they all had a detrimental effect on my self-esteem and sense of self-worth. For the first time in over two years, I was reminded how shame feels.

In one sense, it felt like I'd gone back to square one. My mood was low, and I felt incredibly vulnerable. The painful memories of the accident flooded back to the front of my mind and the happiness I'd found during my time with the people at Project Walk was all but wiped out. I felt like I was a burden on my husband, and I started blaming myself again for being hit by the car. I faced the lowest of lows and all but lost my capacity for self-compassion. Fortunately, there was still part of me that knew it was not only the robotics or the exoskeletons or any of the amazing technology I had access to during my time at Project Walk that helped me with my physical injury – it was self-compassion. So, surely self-compassion could also help me with the challenges in my professional life back in Australia.

Once I started implementing self-compassion in my professional life, I was much less bothered when my boss commented about not being up to date with my knowledge. All I did was study ten times harder than my peers. I decided not to be a lone ranger anymore either. I reached out to my family and close friends for help. I accepted my injury for what it was and accepted myself for just being me. Basically, I didn't allow having fallen behind a bit to hold me back in any way. The result of this new attitude was that I not only managed to pass my fellowship exams in Rehabilitation Medicine in 2014 but I also went on to pass my fellowship exams in Pain Medicine in 2017.

I can genuinely congratulate myself now from a place of self-compassion. It wasn't easy but I built a beautiful life from something traumatic and sad. By 2018, I started working as a pain physician and going home to a rich family life with a thriving three-year-old called Joseph. I literally rose from the ashes and became a formidable force in the lives of my family and friends. I became much more influential around my medical colleagues who had learnt to respect me all the more for the challenges I overcome. Most important of all, I learnt to respect myself. I rebuilt my self-worth through self-compassion and, in the process, became a much more compassionate doctor. I now inspire my patients to transform their lives from misery and self-loathing to a place of deep self-compassion. This enables them to lead better-quality lives, regardless of any illnesses or injuries they might have.

It wasn't all rosy though. Little did I know, I was slowly edging towards burnout again towards the end of 2018. I was exhausted from juggling physical therapy and rehabilitation for my injury with my medical work as a pain physician and my responsibilities as a mother. This combination left me depleted of energy and extremely vulnerable to breaking down or burning out.

The upshot of it was that I developed severe burnout in the middle of 2019. My spinal cord injury, full-time work as a pain physician and motherhood all took their toll on my body. One day, I was so exhausted that I was physically and emotionally incapable of getting out of bed. I was meant to go to work and kept telling myself I needed to get up and get ready for work. Eventually, I managed to transfer myself to my wheelchair, but my brain was in a complete fog of cognitive fatigue. No matter how hard I was trying to be able to show up for my family, my patients and my friends, I wound up having to take two months off work to rest. It took me every bit of that two months to get better physically, but it took a lot longer to rehabilitate myself emotionally, mentally and spiritually.

I decided to hit the books and find out everything I could about burnout. I found out that female doctors have a higher rate of burnout than their male counterparts and that the seven main causes of burnout in female doctors are:

- anxiety (e.g. worrying about things like passing exams or financial issues)
- putting everyone else's needs ahead of our own
- work-related conflict with supervisors or colleagues
- relationship issues with a partner or children
- fear of failure and imposter syndrome
- being overworked, travelling to multiple hospitals every day, working late and working unscheduled overtime
- juggling exams, work and relationships
- traumatic patient stories.

I also learnt that the consequences of burnout when these things are not addressed include:

- constantly elevated cortisol and adrenaline levels
- damaged blood vessels and elevated blood pressure
- heart disease and stroke
- impaired immune system
- auto-immune disease and inflammation

- reduced gut health, which affects the gut-brain axis
- headaches and back pain as a result of chronic tension
- depression
- suicide.

In theory, self-compassion is easy to get a handle on, but it can be significantly harder to implement. Even though I knew the theory well and had experienced the benefits of self-compassion in the past, back in the 'real world' I remained highly self-critical and judgemental. I harboured a harsh inner monologue, keeping my problems, faults and failures at the forefront of my mind. Fortunately, there was a moment of respite from the bully in my head and I remembered all the ways self-compassion had helped me overcome adversities in the past. Intellectually, I knew if I didn't learn to be kind and compassionate towards myself again, I would always struggle to prioritise my wellbeing.

As they say, there are no 'accidents.' Just when I really needed it, a self-compassion writing exercise from *The Mindful Self Compassion Workbook, A proven way to accept yourself, build inner strength and thrive* by Kirsten Neff and Chris Germer, caught my eye. It said:

Begin by thinking of something that makes you feel inadequate or bad about yourself. This could relate to any aspect of your life: your body, work, relationships, habits, skills or anything else. Write down the emotions you feel as you think about this. Then imagine a friend who is unconditionally loving, accepting, kind and compassionate. Imagine this friend can see your strengths, and also your weakness, and does not judge you for them. Think about this friend accepting that you are only human and understanding your life experiences. Write a letter to yourself from the perspective of this imagined friend.

At that point, tears started streaming down my face. I was crying because I was touched by this idea, and I also realised I still had a long way to go in terms of managing the cognitive and emotional aspect of my burnout. I started writing myself a letter from the perspective of a kind and loving friend. Here's what my letter looked like:

Dear Olivia,

I see how much you care about your work, and how much time and effort you put into helping those in your care. I know you blame yourself when the outcome of your efforts are not what you would like them to be. I know how meticulously you look for any mistakes you have made or anywhere you could have done better. What I want you to know is that no matter how perfectly you do your job, or how hard you work, you cannot control everything. As unfortunate as it is, some bad outcomes are inevitable. You need to remember you are only human. Everyone makes mistakes and everyone is imperfect, so you shouldn't worry about not being perfect. Nobody is. What's more, you are the only one who expects you to be that way.

I know it is not easy to change the way you feel about these things and I know you will always care deeply about those around you. But you have to do something to take the pressure off yourself. Do not stay up at night worrying. Have fun with your family! Enjoy BEING in the present moment with your kids! Use your kids' eyes as a mirror to look at yourself differently and see the person that they really love. You are more than your career or the mistakes you have made.

From your loving friend

My journey from burnout to recovery once again started with accepting my struggles, showing myself compassion and facing the fact that I would inevitably have issues in my life. The key to this is to not let having issues and struggles mean we can't strive for wellbeing.

Self-compassion is about increasing our capacity to accept whatever comes our way, rather than resisting it. I realised that if I happen to make a mistake or come up against a roadblock on my journey to recovery, I should not lose heart. I should just keep being kind to myself. And if things don't work out, I can always reassess the situation, try something different and work towards an alternative solution. Everything feels different when we take away the judgement and just let what will be, be.

I learnt that once I developed self-compassion, I had a powerful tool that is a protective mechanism against depression, anxiety and negative emotions like fear, irritability, hostility and distress. I find self-compassion to be particularly helpful when I'm under stress. Stress can arise from many sources: internal, external, physical, mental or emotional. Whatever the catalyst, stress triggers a complex physical response from our neurological and endocrine systems. Specifically, it releases cortisol and adrenaline into our body. These hormones result in an increased heart rate, rapid breathing, muscle tension and sweating. In contrast, self-compassion deactivates our stress response and triggers feelings of warmth and safety by way of the release of a hormone called oxytocin.

Having just started my creative business as a medical entrepreneur in December 2020, I noticed that old paradigms still come back to visit from time to time. I'm much better at not being fazed when things like negative self-talk, self-criticism or self-judgement come up these days, though. Implementing the self-compassion practices that are starting to feel like second nature to me, usually gets me back on track. Sometimes, that involves reading the words I wrote in my journal a little while ago out loud to myself:

Sometimes, I worry that you are unable to see the amazing person you are. I see your kind heart. I see your compassion, empathy, creativity and talent for writing. You are launching your coaching business next month so that you can encourage and uplift your clients. Your mission is to inspire doctors to pursue their dreams and lead the heart-centred lives they deserve. You are writing a book to give your medical peers a voice to honour their struggles and their joys. You've created a following of heart-centred medical entrepreneurs and leaders on Facebook because you have so much value to give. I'm proud of you for showing up for Facebook lives, even though they make you feel sick because you are not used to being in the spotlight.

Self-compassion is not passive or self-indulgent. It is an active process that taps into the basic rights around compassion that all humans deserve. Compassion is not something that has to be earned. We have a right to compassion, even when we feel like we don't deserve it, such as when we make a mistake or feel like a particularly undesirable situation is our fault. Any and all human suffering, regardless of the cause, deserves a kind and compassionate response.

Although applying self-compassion is simple, many people, especially doctors, have trouble doing it. This is hardly surprising when you think about how many years of ingrained patterning we are trying to change.

Self-compassion is the core ingredient of the *heart-centredness of medicine*. To help you to start your journey towards heart-centredness right now, I've included a couple of simple self-compassion exercises for you.

Self-compassion exercises

The following action steps will help you implement self-compassion practices in your personal and professional life, allowing you to thrive at work and at home.

Action 1: Increase awareness

Over the next few days, carry a journal or notebook with you and pay attention to how you react to even the tiniest amount of personal suffering. Jot down anything you notice. It could be a thought you have because you've made a mistake. Or disappointment you feel about not having lived up to your own expectations. Or an emptiness or agitation in your gut because of loneliness, embarrassment, grief, shame and so on. Try to capture the exact words and phrases you say to yourself. Write them down and read back through them a couple of days later to see whether there are any common themes or trends showing up. Does anything surprise you? How do you feel about the way you speak to yourself?

Action 2: How would you treat a friend?

This exercise is based on the work of Dr Kristin Neff and Chris Germer, the people behind a number of fabulous programs on self-compassion. You will need to use your journal again. The first step is to think about a time when a good friend felt bad about themselves or was going through a challenging time. Write down the things you would do or say in that sort of situation, noting the tone of voice you would use.

Then think of a time you've struggled emotionally because you felt bad about yourself. How do you usually respond? What words or tone of voice do you usually use? What actions do you take?

Reflect on the difference between the way you treat yourself and the way you treat others. Why do you think there is a difference?

Now consider what might happen if you responded to yourself in the same way you respond to friends. Write down some thoughts about how this awareness might change the way you feel and behave during difficult times.

Outcome of self-compassion exercises

The awareness you are starting to develop around your inclination towards self-criticism, and how easy it is to flip this tendency and show yourself more kindness, is something you can use to get better at catching self-criticism before it has a chance to undermine your confidence and wellbeing. To take this a step further, you could even carry a letter to the self-critical part of yourself around with you, or memorise a short phrase such as:

I know you are trying to protect me in some way, but it is not helpful right now. I acknowledge the suffering I feel in this moment and I choose to respond to it with kindness and compassion.

Through this conscious effort to change your internal dialogue, you will reduce the amount of cortisol and adrenaline that floods your body when your stress response is triggered by self-criticism. At the same time, you will increase the amount of dopamine in your body through generating positive and compassionate thoughts.

Don't be discouraged if these exercises feel uncomfortable in the beginning. Remember, you've spent your whole life so far being self-critical and it's only reasonable that shifting your internal thought processes may take a bit of time. But I promise you, it is totally worth the effort.

Secret Ingredient Four: Mindfulness
Choosing mindfulness over distraction

Imagine it's 6:30 pm one evening in June 2019. You've just completed a full day of work and your child is trying to get your attention as you walk through the door. You are so distracted by the day's events you don't even hear the story he is telling you about his day at school. He looks disappointed and sad when he realises you're not listening but you don't notice because your mind is totally focused on what you need to do to get ready for tomorrow.

That was me. I used to be so distracted, I missed out on the special bond parents can build with their children through the million and one little moments that offer the opportunity for connection a day-to-day basis. I want you to know that I'm on this journey with you. I am still in the process of breaking the old patterns that were robbing me of so much, including the beautiful connection with my children, and I am now forging through awareness and attention.

Earlier on the same day, at 12:30 pm, I was having my lunch break at the pain clinic where I worked and one of my colleagues came in and interrupted my break to talk about a patient. I was really frustrated at not being able to enjoy my lunch without interruptions after a busy morning seeing complex patients, formulating management plans for them and juggling a number of other things that had come up since I arrived at the clinic. I wound up gulping down my food and swallowing my frustration in a hurry to get back to work so I didn't get further behind than I already felt I was. Not surprisingly, I was both exhausted and wired up with adrenaline when I finished work and was looking forward to going home and seeing my family. Just as I was getting ready to leave, the same colleague came into my office to talk about another patient. I felt my pulse rising. It actually felt as if my blood was starting to boil. Feelings of helplessness, anxiety and frustration all came up for me when I saw my colleague approaching. Impatient thoughts ran through my mind and my inner voice started ranting about the situation. So, I'm expressing it politely when I say I was somewhat less than primed to go home and have quality time with my family.

Now imagine me at 7:30 pm on the same day. I've been home for an hour. The problem is that I wasn't really there. My body was there but my head was still back in the office. I was fully in planning mode as I was feeding my three-year-old son, Joseph, his dinner. I heard the notification sound ping on my iPhone, and I groaned as I grabbed it and looked at my emails. My three-year-old would have been better off trying to show the drawing he had done especially for me to a robot. He certainly wasn't getting through to me, no matter how many times he literally pushed his drawing in my face.

"Mummy, here is my drawing. Mummy … Mummy! You aren't listening to me. Mummy, you don't love me."

Hearing those words was what it took for me to snap out of the twilight zone I was in. Looking back on this now, I have to say I'm grateful for the incredible mother's guilt I felt in that moment because it was the catalyst for me to change before it was too late.

You probably haven't noticed it, but we take a lot of mental shortcuts with the routines we have in place. For example, family life is really repetitive: make dinner, clear the table, do the dishes, get the kids in the bath and into bed, get ready for bed yourself. These routines help us get through our busy life but the downside is that we can lose our ability to see things as they really are when we are sleepwalking through the routines of our life. What's more, we often walk around all day with our heads stuck in a screen. We don't take a moment to look up and appreciate the beautiful sky, or the roses blooming in the garden, or the beautiful child in the highchair wanting to give us a drawing he has been waiting all day to show us. What's worse, we miss out on vicariously enjoying the wonderful sense of curiosity children naturally bring to the world around them.

In fact, we miss out on so much when we spend most of our time with our children on autopilot. Our minds are fixed on accomplishing goals, solving problems, planning and strategising how we're going to do everything we have to get done day after day.

If we are not fully present with our kids, we miss the chance to become attuned with their cues that give us an opportunity to understand what's happening for them under the surface. We might miss the signal that our child needs a hug or help of some kind. Whereas, if we can be mindful, we will be in a much better position to offer our children the thoughtful, empathetic responses they need.

What I want you to know is that you are not a bad person if you are inclined to be reactive rather than mindful. The thing is that reactions just happen. We are not choosing to turn on our frustrated thoughts, helpless feelings or our physiological stress reaction. We are simply reacting in the moment when we are operating on autopilot. The thing to know about stress is that it activates the prehistoric part of our brain called the limbic system.

This means we literally cannot access the rational part of our brain, the prefrontal cortex, when our stress response is triggered.

What can we do about this? Thankfully, there is a time-tested intervention called mindfulness meditation that will save the day. As Jon Kabat-Zinn, well-known author and founder of the Stress Reduction Clinic at the University of Massachusetts says, mindfulness is the 'awareness that arises through paying attention on purpose, in the present moment and non-judgementally.' Research has shown that mindfulness can help reduce stress, depression and anxiety. It increases our energy levels, improves our memory and sharpens our concentration. It is also incredibly helpful for anyone who needs help falling asleep at night or with pain management. Meditation is not just something that alternative thinkers do. It is literally the practice of training the mind to become less reactive and more present. Mindfulness meditation is about intentionally training our attention to be in the present moment, non-reactive and non-judgementally curious.

The amazing thing is that mindfulness meditation actually changes the shape of our brain. It shrinks the part of the brain that's responsible for the fight or flight response (the amygdala) and thickens the prefrontal cortex, which is responsible for all our executive functions, like decision-making and the ability to solve problems. This means that through mindfulness meditation, we can predispose ourselves to respond in a thoughtful and constructive way to the things that happen on a day-to-day basis, rather than a reactive, and possibly destructive, way.

As we start to practise mindfulness, essentially bringing our attention into the present moment with kindness and curiosity, we can watch the ripple effect of bringing that awareness, kindness and curiosity to the lives of our children and the other people we interact with. I will be forever grateful to the circumstances that brought my mindfulness meditation teacher, Chibs Orereke, into my life. We started with short meditation practices. This was extremely useful for me on a practical level because I only had pockets of time to invest in getting my life back on track. It turned out that this was fine because research shows a short meditation practice is the gold standard for reducing reactivity.

Just because the effect of mindfulness meditation is profound doesn't mean bringing it about has to be complicated. It's as simple as choosing a regular time each day to establish the habit of sitting in a quiet place to meditate. It's best if you sit in an upright but relaxed pose on a chair or cushion. Gently close your eyes as you bring your attention to your breath and your body. Expect your mind to wander; that is normal and nothing to worry about. Whatever you do, don't let thoughts popping into your mind convince you that you're not doing it properly. The goal is not to stop your thoughts, but to train your attention. The aim is to spend more time in the present moment and less time lost in distraction.

I remember listening to a podcast featuring Dr Dan Siegel, a clinical professor of psychiatry, an author and an expert on attachment, mindfulness and the brain. In the podcast, he said, "parental presence is key to optimising the chance of your child having a life of wellbeing and resilience."

It sounds amazing, right? But let's be real here: no one is ever going to be a hundred per cent present. And you know what – it doesn't matter. This is about taking the middle path. It's about using the tools of mindfulness to become more present for our children and reducing our predisposition to default to the stress response. Being a present parent means really seeing, hearing and understanding what's going on for them. It means letting go of our agenda and preconceived notions and, instead, being curious about what 'just is.' Your meditation practice will help you to become more present for your child and yourself. It will also enable you to see your child with the fresh eyes of 'the beginner's mind.' This Zen Buddhist practice can help us to calm our reactivity and see life as a beginner does, where every situation is a learning opportunity.

The beginner's mind is about bringing a 'freshness' to each moment. I'd love for you to try the following practice this week to see how it feels to start to take control of your state. All things being equal, this should help you to get out of autopilot mode, to let go of preconceived notions and move into a place of presence and curiosity. Remember, the beauty of neuroplasticity is that whatever we practise becomes stronger.

When we slow down and live more mindfully with awareness in the present moment, we get to see the richness of the world around us. Savouring and appreciating the world not only feels good, but it also lowers our stress levels and helps us to see our problems more clearly and less judgementally.

So, let's practise *Beginner's Mind on a Walk*. Start by seeing the activity of walking with fresh eyes, as if you haven't done it thousands of times already and you don't know what to expect. Really *look* into the path. Notice the trees, the concrete, the buildings and the landscape. Try to see the kinds of details you might not normally notice. Really get a sense of the textures, tastes, smells and appearance of the world around you. Pay close attention and see what happens.

Secret Ingredient Five: Belonging

This is a big topic to cover, so I've broken this chapter down into two parts.

Part One: Choosing connectedness over loneliness

Burnout can be such a lonely journey. I pretended everything was alright every single day when I turned up for work in a burnt-out state in 2019. The clinic was relentless and the workload endless. Somehow, I found the will to push through all my duties, even though I was exhausted and emotionally drained by the end of each and every day. The same cycle happened the next day and the day after that. I was like a zombie teetering on a precipice.

The more burnt out I was, the more socially withdrawn I became. I felt incredibly lonely, even though I was constantly surrounded by people. This is a common symptom of burnout. It can happen for several reasons, such as:

- being exhausted and having limited energy or motivation for social engagements
- being emotionally drained, making it difficult to deal with feelings and thoughts about others, leading to a loss of empathy

- becoming more easily irritated and frustrated, making relationships tense and less fulfilling
- experiencing feelings of personal inadequacy, which can lead to a loss of confidence both inside and outside the workplace.

As a physician, I know it is easier to manage illness during the early stages, rather than waiting until it's a full-blown outbreak of whatever it is you are facing. Sadly, I know the long list of the late signs of burnout from firsthand experience – insomnia, depression, migraines, gastrointestinal symptoms, relationship problems and a whole lot more. As doctors, we know early signs are harder to detect, so it takes vigilance and awareness to nip things in the bud. Not to mention the fact that doctors are doubly at risk of not recognising these early signs in themselves because of the culture of stoicism that exists within the medical profession. Most doctors I know think stress is just a normal part of the job. They are notorious for holding off on seeking care and they are vulnerable to resorting to the trap of self-medication.

I wish I had done something about the early warning signs of burnout that were right in front of my eyes. In retrospect, I can see they were there in 2017 when I finished the exams I had to sit for my pain fellowship. I remember the feeling of real fatigue that I experienced at the prospect of going to work. Little did I know, my ability to recover was reducing with every day that passed without taking action to deal with the burnout. The following year, 2018, was a blur. It was too late for me to rehabilitate myself without professional help by the time I saw my GP about my problems in July 2019.

We know humans are complex and relationships can be tricky, so it comes as no surprise when creating and sustaining a positive relationship turns out to be harder than we thought it would be. Among other things, we need to be wise to the fact that relationships are a mixed bag and will change over time. They often run the gamut of close bonding moments, disagreements, hurt, disappointment, fun and joy. Some relationships go the distance and others end prematurely. The truth of it is that people can grow apart. This can happen for a multitude of reasons that don't necessarily have anything to do with us as individuals.

I want to encourage you not to let challenges within friendships put you off. This might sound like a funny thing to say but it's worth not taking anything too personally. Friendships and connectedness can bring great joy and they can also bring great pain. One thing I can say for myself, as I look back on my life so far, is I've tended to throw myself in, boots and all. I've allowed myself to experience the highs of love and the joy of friendship, as well as the lows of loss, hurt, disappointment and frustration. I've tried not to let the fear of hurt and loss deter me from investing in relationships and to be grateful for them, even if they feel difficult at times.

I seem to have unconsciously closed ranks and developed a smaller number of close friends since graduating from medical school. Rather than maintaining the larger group of people I socialised with while I was studying, these days I really look forward to regular catch-ups with a small group of close friends who are also doctors. However, during the months leading up to my burnout, I found myself avoiding catching up with even my closest friends. I was actually making up excuses for not being able to go out. My friends seemed to irritate me more than usual and I couldn't muster the emotional energy to be supportive when they were having a hard time. On the rare occasion when I did go out, I was caught in a tug-of-war with myself. I didn't want to tell my friends about what I was going through but dreaded having to put on a 'happy face' and pretend everything was okay.

One thing I definitely learnt through my experience of burnout is that having strong relationships in place is a powerful strategy when it comes to maintaining our health and dealing with difficulties around it. The way I see it, healthy relationships have an overwhelmingly positive impact on our mental and physical wellbeing. The impact comes from both the comfort they provide on an emotional level and in terms of the benefits of the dopamine that is generated by positive relationships. I certainly recognise that whenever I was facing challenges, having solid and genuine relationships in place helped me to cope. Knowing that someone has my back enables me to process emotions better and recover more quickly.

After I got some professional support with my burnout, I slowly started to see my friends again. It took a lot of effort to begin with, but after a while the connections started to feel more natural and enjoyable. I dug deep and bravely shared with my friends what I'd been through. To my surprise, it turned out they had all been through something similar themselves. This shared experience became the glue that strengthened our bond. These friends became part of my support network as I continued to recover and enjoy life again.

My husband, John, was my rock as I clawed my way out of burnout. I saw the look of despair and helplessness on his face as he watched me suffer. The thing is – he wasn't helpless. His presence and his commitment to me were a great help and are an enduring comfort to me. My focus was on strengthening my current relationships with my loved ones and friends and, on a few occasions, forming new ones. I didn't need a plethora of friends. I just needed a small number of strong relationships that were consistent and could be relied upon. These kinds of relationships are invaluable. They provided me with people to reach out to whenever I felt lonely; to share exciting news with; to talk through big decisions with; to laugh with; and to have interesting conversations with. Strong relationships are more than just what people can offer me. They are very much about what I can offer them.

I'd like you to take a moment to think about the state of your relationships right now. The people you are in a relationship with might be friends, family or someone you have a romantic attachment with. Perhaps you have lots of friends, but you don't feel particularly close to any of them. Maybe you feel like you have close work friends but those friendship are only situational. Perhaps you have close friendships that you want to strengthen. Or maybe, at this point in your life, you don't feel like you have any close relationships at all.

Whatever your situation is, there are things you can easily do to help find meaningful relationships or strengthen existing ones. As you read through the two action steps I've included for you here, I want you to consider how they might work for you or whether there is something else you could do instead.

Action step one: reach out

As I mentioned earlier, one of the challenges I struggled with when I was burnt out was engaging in relationships. I was concerned my diminished state left me with very little to offer as a friend. Basically, I felt like I was uninteresting and no fun at all. The truth of it was I was easily irritated and was finding it difficult to muster the emotional energy to deal with other people's energy.

At the same time, I was feeling lonely and isolated, so I got up the gumption to get out of my comfort zone and contacted a close friend called Martha with the view to inviting her to catch up over a coffee. The thing is, I had been waiting for other people to make contact. That didn't work and it actually exacerbated my feelings of loneliness. Martha's response when I reached out to her reminded me that, in reality, other people were probably waiting to be contacted just like I was and would be delighted to catch up if someone reached out to them. I can't tell you how much it meant to me to share my war stories about burnout with Martha, and to support her by listening to hers.

I really want to encourage you to reach out and contact someone. Make a plan to catch up soon and spend some quality time together. If you feel up to it, it would be worth talking about how you're feeling. Opening up about our difficulties can be hard, especially if we usually take the role of supporting others, but you owe it to yourself to break that pattern and allow someone to support you back.

You may find it helpful to prepare for a catch-up by thinking about things you could share and also things you could ask the other person about. Planning beforehand may feel a bit artificial but if you are burnt out, any level of social interaction can feel really difficult – doing a bit of planning might help.

Action step two: join a community group or hobby group

I came across a wide range of options when I was thinking about what I could do to become more connected. There were sporting groups, craft groups, courses on everything from learning to dance to learning another language, and a plethora of options for volunteering. The kind of engagement that happens in these contexts takes away the pressure to 'actively' socialise all the time. Lulls in conversation are easily dealt with by participation in the activity itself, so there's no need to worry about awkward silences. What's more, the fact that everyone involved has an interest in the activity in question provides common ground and a starting point for connection and conversation.

For my part, I joined a book club. It not only gave me great joy, but it also took the pressure off me in terms of having to think about topics of conversation.

I recommend you don't go overboard by offering to organise a group yourself. I say that because it's hard to cancel at the last minute if you need to and, if you're anything like I was, you don't need the extra worry of letting people down if you can't turn up. Or you might even hesitate to make plans for a get-together in the first place for fear that your fluctuating symptoms could flare up. If you do wind up organising a group, though, and you find yourself needing to pull out, do not worry – it's not the end of the world. If you feel comfortable, I'd encourage you to try being open about why you had to cancel. People are usually very understanding and sharing your reasons could be an opportunity to spread awareness of how you and others are affected by burnout. It could also potentially open up avenues of discussion in which other people feel comfortable about sharing their own issues.

Because the solution to loneliness is connectedness, it will be well worth the effort to foster strong relationships. If you do, the world will no longer be such a lonely place for you.

Part Two: Choosing togetherness over disconnection

Disconnection is defined as the energy that is generated when people don't feel seen, heard and valued; they give and receive with judgement; and they are unable to derive sustenance and strength from their relationships.

It's a hard truth but the fact is that, in the digital age we live in, we are simultaneously disconnected while having more access to each other than ever before. We felt alone prior to COVID-19 because, for the most part, we had been using our technology in a way that surrounded us with surface-level connections. The analogy that comes up for me here is that it's like standing by yourself at a party, made up to the nines, looking around at all the guests and still feeling hauntingly alone. My greatest soothing balm during this pandemic has been seeing virtual connections deepening and our devices being used to engage with those we love in a way that is fostering real engagement. I know I am not alone in hoping this continues well into our new normal.

This question of connection matters a lot. A plethora of studies exist, confirming that the people who live longer are those who feel more connected to their community. Dr Lisa Berkman of the Harvard School of Health Sciences observed a group of 7000 people over nine years. Her results showed that those who lacked quality social or community connections, were three times more likely to die of medical illness than those with strong social ties. Other studies show that loneliness is more deadly than obesity and smoking. This is how important our human connections are.

Malcolm Gladwell's book, *Outliers*, opens by looking at the Sicilian-American village of Roseto. This is a place with a notable lack of suicides, alcoholism, drug addiction and crime. Studies have shown that these statistics are the direct result of human connection. Here is an extract from the study featured in Gladwell's book:

They looked at how the Rosetans visited one another, stopping to chat in Italian on the street, say or cooking for one another in their backyards. They learned about the extended family clans that underlay the town's social structure. They saw how many homes had three generations living under one roof ... They counted twenty-two civic organisations in a town of just under two thousand people ... In transplanting the Paesani culture of Southern Italy to the hills of Eastern Pennsylvania, the Rosetans had created a powerful, protective social structure capable of insulating themselves from the pressures of the modern world.

To cut a long story short, human connection is good for your health. I would argue that the world needs things that promote good health now more than ever before. I think we should be talking about how we can replicate the social interactions of a village like Roseto in this era of COVID-19 and ask how we can digitally replicate this feeling of connection at a time when a handshake could be deadly?

I pose this question because I believe it is possible to connect authentically through digital mediums. Interestingly, I felt more connected to people in the virtual world when I was feeling really disconnected from my life during the period I was getting used to my situation after the accident. It took me a long time to reconnect with myself, so it was comforting to be able to be immersed in the world of ideas with the influencers, speakers, podcasters, TEDx speakers, coaches and authors I met on webinars and online forums. These people gave me the sense I was not on my own.

The bottom line is that human beings are wired for connection. From the time we are born to the day we die, we need connection to thrive emotionally, physically, spiritually and intellectually. A decade ago, the idea that we are wired for connection might have been perceived as touchy-feely or New Age thinking. Today, we know the need for connection is more than a feeling or a hunch. It's hard science – neuroscience, to be exact.

In an excerpt of his book, *Social Intelligence: The New Science of Human Relationships*, published in 2007, Daniel Goleman explores how the latest findings in biology and neuroscience confirm that our relationships shape our biology as well as our experiences. As Goleman writes:

Even our most routine encounters act as regulators in the brain, priming our emotions, some desirable, others not. The more strongly connected we are with someone emotionally, the greater the mutual force.

Our innate need for connection makes the consequences of disconnection that much more real and dangerous. The problem is that sometimes we only think we are connected. I say this because technology has become a kind of imposter, making us believe we are connected when we really aren't, at least not in the ways we need to be. In our technology-crazed world, we've confused being communicative with feeling connected. Just because we are plugged in, it doesn't mean our deep need to feel seen and heard is being met. In fact, it could mean exactly the opposite. The reality of hyper-communication is that many people spend more time on Facebook than they do interacting face-to-face with 'real' people. I cannot tell you how many times I've walked into a restaurant and seen two parents on their mobile phones while their kids are busy texting or playing video games on their own devices. It makes me wonder what the point of sitting together is under these circumstances.

As we think about the definition of connection, and how easy it is to mistake our interactions with technology as connecting, we also need to consider letting go of the myth of self-sufficiency. One of the greatest barriers to connection is the importance we place on the idea of 'going it alone.' I see this a lot in medicine, with doctors keeping to themselves and striving to be independent and autonomous. What I find is that many of us are willing to extend a helping hand, but most of us are reluctant to reach out for help when we need it. It's as if we've divided the world into 'those who offer help' and 'those who need help.' The truth is that everyone deserves to be able to move between both of these categories.

Until we can receive with an open heart, we are never really able to give with an open heart either. When we attach judgement to receiving help, we are unknowingly attaching judgement to giving help as well.

I desperately needed help when I was struggling with stress and mental fatigue from burnout in 2019. I needed support, handholding and advice like never before. Turning to my husband, John, my younger brother, William, and my wonderful friends shifted the relationship I had with these people in a really positive way. Our esteem and love deepened when I gave myself permission to fall apart and be imperfect, and to accept the strength and incredible wisdom my special connections openly shared with me. If connection is the energy that surges between people, we have to remember that those surges are meant to travel in both directions.

So, what is togetherness? It is much more than sharing the same physical space. It is the pleasant feeling of being united with other people in friendship and understanding. When people are together, they connect physically. When people are in togetherness, they share the energy of being mentally and emotionally connected. When we are connected in this way, we share a spiritual partnership.

Whereas, when we are together in separateness, we are co-dependently sharing the same space but leading our own lives though different realities.

I developed beautiful friendships with the other clients at the Project Walk Paralysis Recovery Centre in San Diego. We were connected through one common thread – spinal cord injury.

Those friendships have endured, even though we are now located in different parts of the world.

In January 2021, when I was feeling centred and inspired to make a difference, I formed my own Facebook group called *The Heart-Centred Medical Female Entrepreneurs and Leaders*. As I'm writing now, there are 463 members who are sharing their experiences, including various degrees of burnout. What I'm hearing in the group matches the sentiments of my coaching clients, who are mainly female doctors.

The common experiences of burnout that I've distilled from the numerous conversations I've had in this space are:
- often feeling overwhelmed and full of self-doubt
- being angry about the way the healthcare system overworks doctors
- feeling guilty about not spending enough time with their partner or children
- beating themselves up for not setting effective boundaries
- feeling trapped and helpless in a space where life is out of balance
- realising they've bought into a life that is 'prestigious, yet empty'
- feeling ripped off because the reality of being a doctor does not live up to their expectations
- feeling powerless to stop hurtling towards a cliff that they're afraid of falling off.

I talk to a lot of female doctors who tell me they are exhausted and overwhelmed and just too busy to do a self-help program or anything like that. This breaks my heart because, after coming out the other end of burnout myself, I know it doesn't have to be this way. In my *Life Transformation for Doctors* program, I coach and mentor female doctors who have had enough. Those who take the first step of picking up the phone and having a conversation with me don't realise the potential for the massive transformation they are opening themselves up to. They certainly know it when it happens though. For example, Dr Lily went from feeling stressed, overwhelmed and anxious, to having clarity, confidence and certainty in her life. She told me that, for the first time in a very long time, she felt supported, valued and recognised for her contribution at work and at home. The biggest deal of all is that Dr Lily now recognises her own value and self-worth and has the skills and courage to demand a fair go. The dynamics in her life are completely changed. They are aligned with her wellbeing, and never again will she forget to put the oxygen mask on herself first.

Dr Amanda's journey was one of self-discovery and re-awakening. She is now revelling in the fact that she is more relaxed, more empowered and even able to breathe more easily. Dr Amanda is equipped with the self-compassion tools she needs to maintain the improvements she made in all aspects of her life through doing my program. With her physical and emotional wellbeing restored, Dr Amanda is ready to be seen, to share her truth and to make a big impact on the lives of others.

I feel incredibly proud to have started a movement with doctors from all over the world. We are on a mission to end physician burnout. The African proverb, 'If you want to go fast, go alone. If you want to go far, go together' rings totally true to me.

Secret Ingredient Six: Vulnerability
Choosing vulnerability over controlling self and others

Controlling oneself and others comes from a worldview based around the idea of winning and losing. It is the default strategy that a lot of people use to avoid feeling vulnerable. The only problem is – it doesn't work.

I interviewed many doctors in the process of writing this book. One of the things I asked them to do was describe what makes them feel vulnerable. These are a few of the answers I got:

- Admitting to the first medical error I made during my internship days.
- Apologising to a nursing colleague about how I spoke to her during a clinical handover.
- Giving feedback to a junior medical staff member who was underperforming.
- Getting feedback from a senior medical staff member.

Vulnerable experiences are not easy to bear because they make us feel uncertain and anxious. In most cases, they make us go into self-protection mode. Some of us show up with courage, some of us shrink and go into hiding, some of us thrash about and try to deflect the discomfort by placing blame, criticising, being cynical or fearmongering.

How should we position ourselves in relation to vulnerability? If we shield ourselves from all feedback and disconnect from our feelings, we stop growing. On the other hand, we can increase our capacity to deal with discomfort if we engage with the feedback that comes our way by honestly looking at it to see if there is anything we can take from it as a way of learning how to do something better.

The problem with disconnecting from our feelings is that sealing off our heart doesn't just stop us from feeling hurt, it also stops us from feeling love.

To be clear, vulnerability is the feeling we experience during times of uncertainty, risk and emotional exposure. Here are my observations of how doctors feel about vulnerability:

I don't do vulnerability

Our daily lives are full of uncertainty, risk and emotional exposure. This is especially the case in medicine. Not 'doing vulnerability' is not really an option. However, a lot of doctors say they don't do vulnerability because they perceive it as a sign of weakness or a flaw in their character. Pretending, and actually believing, they don't do vulnerability means they are letting fear control their thinking and behaviour. This often leads to acting out or shutting down.

Ask yourself, "How do I act when I am feeling vulnerable?" If you are coming from a place of awareness, you might recognise that you sometimes go into avoidance or denial when you feel vulnerable, and sometimes you take a deep breath and silently tell yourself that you're okay as you walk into your boss' office knowing you're going to get a grilling (or something like that).

One thing I want to say is that if you've decided to skip over this question – and I know I would have back in the day – chances are that you might really benefit from not skipping over it and honestly assessing where you're positioned when it comes to gaining strength in your vulnerability, rather than weakness through avoiding it.

I can go it alone

Some doctors tell me they don't need to be vulnerable because they are perfectly capable of handling whatever life throws at them (i.e. they don't need anyone's help). I know where they're coming from. Some days, I wish I could just put my head down and do what I need to do without involving anyone else. The problem is that going through life as if you don't need anyone pushes against everything it means to be human. It goes against everything we know about human neurobiology because we are literally hardwired for connection. From our mirror neurons to language, we are a social species and we suffer greatly in the absence of authentic connection. Authentic connection does not require us to be hustling for acceptance or changing who we are to fit in. It just requires us to turn up as we really are.

Connection with others is not only good from the touchy-feely point of view. We also derive strength from our collective ability to plan, communicate and work together. The bottom line is that our neural, hormonal and genetic make-up supports interdependence over independence one hundred per cent of the time.

How do I know if I can trust someone enough to be vulnerable around them?

Medicine can be a stressful and hard-core environment to work in. Most doctors think that if they are stupid enough to let someone know their vulnerabilities, it's just a matter of time before someone will use that against them. I hate to say it, but this is a valid concern. There have been cases where doctors with mental health issues have told their colleagues about their struggles, only to find these same colleagues either reporting them to the head of their department or their governing medical bodies. This then sets off a whirlwind of stressful and anxiety-provoking times, where the person who took the risk and opened their heart feels betrayed and even more vulnerable than they were before.

Notwithstanding the importance of listening to our gut so we don't wind up in trouble we could have avoided, we need to have a modicum of trust to feel safe enough to show vulnerability. We need to be vulnerable in order to build trust. The building of trust is a slow, iterative and layered process that happens over time. Trusting and being vulnerable both involve risk – that's what makes them such courageous and rare commodities in the world we live in.

I've found, from firsthand experience, that trust is built through seemingly inconsequential 'sliding door' moments. On the University of California, Berkeley's *Greater Good* website, John Gottman gives a relevant example of the way trust-building plays out in his relationship with his wife. He shares what happened one night when he really wanted to finish a novel he was reading. At one point, he put the novel on his bedside table and walked into the bathroom. As he entered, he saw his wife's face reflected in the mirror. He noticed she looked sad as she was brushing her hair. That was a sliding door moment because he recognised he had a choice. He could have snuck out of the bathroom to avoid opening the can of worms around his wife's sadness that night. Instead, in line with the fact he is a sensitive researcher of relationships, he decided to take the brush from her hand and ask her tenderly why she was sad. She then told him what was going on for her and he comforted her. Gottman described this as a situation where trust was built in the very moment he decided not to turn away.

One moment like this may not be all that important in the scheme of things but if you are always choosing to turn away, trust will erode and the degree of genuine connection that exists within the relationship will be slowly watered down. Essentially, trust is the stacking and layering of small moments and the sharing of vulnerability over time. Trust and vulnerability grow together. To betray one is to destroy both.

Vulnerability involves disclosing my personal and professional weaknesses and it will compromise my position as a leader

I am not a proponent of oversharing, the indiscriminate disclosure of information as a leadership tool or vulnerability for its own sake. But I strongly feel that, without being prepared to be vulnerable, we cannot be courageous leaders.

Psychological safety is the state where team members feel safe to take risks and be vulnerable with each other. As clinical leaders, we can build trust by naming unsaid emotions and creating what we call a 'safe container.' One way to show real leadership is by asking team members what they need to feel open and safe within team discussions. This is one of the easiest practices to implement and you'll be surprised at the return you get in terms of trust-building and improving the quality of feedback and conversations that take place within the team. It's a shame this kind of approach is rarely seen in the medical field. Instead, the things that frequently show up and act as a barrier to psychological safety include judgement, the giving of unsolicited advice, interrupting and not respecting the importance of keeping whatever is said within the group.

Harvard Business School Professor, Amy Edmondson, coined the phrase 'psychological safety.' In her book, *Teaming*, she writes:

Simply put, psychological safety makes it possible to give tough feedback and have difficult conversations without the need to tiptoe around the truth.

In psychologically safe environments, people believe that if they make a mistake, others will not penalise them or think less of them for it. They also believe that others will not resent or humiliate them when they ask for help. This belief comes about when people both trust and respect each other, and it produces a sense of confidence that the group will not embarrass, reject or punish someone for speaking up. Thus, psychological safety is a taken-for-granted belief about how others will respond when you ask a question, seek feedback, admit a mistake or propose a possibly wacky idea.

Most people feel a need to 'manage' interpersonal risk to retain a good image, especially at work and even more so in the presence of those who are in the position of formally evaluating their performance. This need is both instrumental (in the sense that promotions and rewards may depend on the impressions held by bosses and others about us) and socio-emotional (because we simply prefer approval over disapproval).

Psychological safety does not imply a cosy situation in which people are necessarily friends. Nor does it suggest an absence of pressure or problems. The behaviours that people need from their team or group to feel psychologically safe almost always include listening, staying curious, being honest and keeping confidences.

I've seen a couple of leaders in medicine who have been honest about their struggles, staying calm while naming the anxiety they have and explaining how it has been showing up for them. They are self-aware and regularly check in with themselves, as well as asking the team what support looks like for them. What I appreciate about this particular approach is that it not only offers the opportunity for clarity, and sets the team up for success, but asking people for specific examples of what supportive behaviours look like to them has a double-barrelled effect by holding them accountable for asking for what they need.

When you put this approach into practice, don't be surprised if you see people struggling to come up with examples of supportive behaviours. That's because we are not accustomed to asking for exactly what we need. Paradoxically, we then often feel resentful or disappointed when we don't get it. It's a sad indictment that most of us can tell you what support doesn't look like much more easily than what it does look like. Over time, this practice of asking people to verbalise what they need will be a huge confidence booster as well as building trust and respect.

Secret Ingredient Seven: Gratitude
Choosing gratitude over feeling ungrateful

Gratitude can be a vulnerable and intense experience. We are an anxious people and many of us have very little tolerance for vulnerability. The thing I want to mention here is that our anxiety and fear come from a place of scarcity, whereas gratitude comes from a place of abundance.

In the healthcare industry I hear people say things that reflect the fact they are coming from a place of scarcity all the time. The kinds of things I'm talking about here are:

- I am not going to allow myself to feel this joy because I know it will not last.
- Acknowledging how grateful I am is an invitation for disaster.
- How can I be grateful when I see so much trauma, pain and suffering around me?
- I am not going to be grateful for the success around me as I deserve more and I want to be externally validated by my boss, my fellow medical colleagues and so on before gratitude is appropriate.
- I am not grateful for my current achievements because I am such a competent and intelligent doctor that I deserve to be put on a pedestal by others.

I'm a person who's been prone to worry my whole life. Becoming a mother took this tendency to a whole other level. Negotiating joy, gratitude and scarcity all at the same time felt like a full-time job. For years, my fear of something terrible happening to my children actually prevented me from fully embracing the joy and gratitude that having them in my life opened up for me. Every time I came too close to relaxing into sheer joyfulness about my children and my love for them, the thought of something terrible happening would pop into my mind. It wasn't uncommon for me to get a picture of losing everything in a flash. For example, as a medical mother, I used to find myself regularly catastrophising about worst case scenarios whenever my children got sick or hurt themselves in some way. As we know, knowledge can be a blessing and a curse.

During the pandemic in 2020, I mustered the courage to approach a mindset coach so I could work on my anxiety, overwhelm and stress and make some room for gratitude to rear its head. As we started to peel back the layers, I realised that my 'too good to be true' thinking was totally related to fear, scarcity and vulnerability. Realising that those are pretty universal emotions, I gathered the courage to talk about my anxiety with my family, friends and colleagues. In fact, I shared a classic example of standing over my son watching him sleep, feeling totally engulfed in gratitude, then being ripped out of that joyful moment by images of something bad happening to him. It turns out that I am not alone here. Once I opened the Pandora's box of the plethora of hideous prospects my imagination had thrown up for me, all of my medical mums and my non-medical friends who have kids started relaying similar experiences.

Most of us have experienced being on the edge of joy, only to be overcome by feelings of vulnerability. This happens because intense feelings of love will often bring up the fear of loss. The trick is to be able to transform vulnerability into gratitude. Brené Brown sums it up beautifully when she says, "The dark does not destroy the light; it defines it. It is our fear of the dark that casts our joy into the shadows."

There's no question that these can be seen as anxious and fearful times we live in. We can choose to live in that space and see the world through the filter of scarcity, or we can choose to live in a space that allows for both vulnerability and trust. That's a space where gratitude and love can be felt more freely. Even the most aware of us are apt to feel afraid of losing what we love the most in moments of stress. We hate the fact there are no guarantees and we think that not being grateful and not feeling joy will make it hurt less when the things we fear losing aren't there anymore. This is the vicious cycle of scarcity and uncertainty. We think if we can beat vulnerability to the punch by imagining loss, we will suffer less. The truth is that this is completely wrong. It is also wrong to think there are no guarantees. There is actually one guarantee – if we are not practising gratitude and allowing ourselves to feel joy, we are missing out on the things that have the power to sustain us during the inevitable hard times. These are the same things that have the power to absolutely light us up when times are good.

Gratitude is a spiritual practice that is bound to a belief in human interconnectedness and a power greater than ourselves. It seems that gratitude without practice may be like faith without belief – it does not exist.

Gratitude is a bit of a buzzword and sometimes comes across sounding a little bit too simple and too good to be true. In fact, gratitude is simply the act of deliberately focusing our mind on things we feel grateful for. Just because it sounds simple doesn't mean it's not powerful. There is actually a lot at stake here. Research shows that gratitude can actually make people happier, improve their mood, improve depressive symptoms and make relationships more satisfying. This is because deliberately focusing on the things we are grateful for will create or strengthen the positive neural pathways in our brain. In fact, gratitude can be a useful tool for retraining our brains to be more positive, which helps us to live more satisfying and happy lives.

The good news is that regular gratitude exercises can be easily incorporated into your life, and you can choose from a multitude of approaches to find the one that suits you best. You might like to practise gratitude every day, or less frequently.

I will forever be grateful to gratitude because it played a big part in my recovery from my spinal cord injury. I'm now in a position to be grateful for the accident that caused the injury because it taught me resilience, tenacity and inner strength. I am also incredibly grateful to my trainers at the Project Walk Paralysis Recovery Centre in San Diego, as well as my physiotherapist in Melbourne. Most important of all is the immense gratitude for my husband, John, who continues to stand by me in times of sadness, sorrow and fear. I also owe a debt of gratitude to my brothers, William and Andrew, and my parents, Daniel and Agnes. I can't thank you enough for standing by my side through all my painful years.

As far as my own practice around gratitude goes, I can report that I've been keeping a couple of gratitude journals for three years, as well as doing daily gratitude meditations and prayers and even stopping during my stressful days at the hospital to actually say these words out loud: "I am grateful for …" Perhaps the most important thing of all is that I've let go of perfectionism and I don't beat myself up if I ever find I'm falling out of these habits that have been sustaining me. All I do is remember how my stressed-out life used to feel, do a meditation and move on.

These might sound like simple little things that couldn't really make much difference but I promise you they can and they do. I'm not only speaking for myself here. My clients often tell me how much difference stopping to be grateful throughout their day has made to their life.

Here are some things you could consider doing to help bring more gratitude into your life.

- Each night, before going to bed, write down three things you are grateful for.
- Once a week, spend ten minutes writing in depth about one or two things you feel grateful for.
- Every night, around the dinner table, share with your family something you are grateful for.
- If you pray, express gratitude in your prayers.
- Communicate gratitude towards others through letters, cards, emails, texts or by just telling them how you feel about them.

It doesn't matter exactly what you express gratitude for. It can be something profound or something quite mundane. Don't be fooled into thinking you need to start lots of gratitude exercises at once to get any effect. It's far better to choose one thing that resonates with you and stick to it regularly for several months, rather than starting lots of exercises and then giving up because you feel overwhelmed about having to do all of them every day.

Each time you experience fear or a sense of scarcity, I want you to try to call forward joy and sufficiency by acknowledging the fear, then transforming it into gratitude. Saying the following sentences out loud will help: "I am feeling vulnerable. That is okay. I am so grateful for …" I can put my hand on my heart as I tell you that doing this has absolutely increased my capacity for joy and changed my life completely.

We are all unique and different strategies will work differently for different people. So please don't give up if you try something and find it doesn't really help. You can either let that practice go and try something different or seek some professional advice to support you to set up a practice that will enable you to experience more joy in your life through gratitude.

Secret Ingredient Eight: Energised
Choosing being energised over being stressed

Millions of people around the globe found their world tipped upside down when the COVID-19 pandemic struck. Many had to make a sudden transition to working remotely. Not surprisingly, some employers worried about maintaining employee productivity. I certainly don't begrudge that, but what they should also have been concerned about was a longer-term risk – employee burnout.

The risk was, and still is, substantial and real. The lines between work and non-work are blurring in new and unusual ways. For example, many employees who are working remotely for the first time are likely to struggle to preserve healthy boundaries between their professional and personal lives. To signal their loyalty and productivity, many feel like they have to be working all the time. Afternoons will blend with evenings; weekdays will blend with weekends; and the idea of time off starts to seem kind of old-fashioned. Meanwhile, the upside of working remotely is that people are saving a lot of time because they don't have to commute to and from a workplace. What's more, businesses are saving a lot of money on rent they would otherwise be paying for a workplace that is no longer needed. The upshot of this is that even when Covid is a thing of the past, some employees may be asked to continue working remotely, or they themselves might put in a request to continue to work from home instead of going back into the office every day.

I was working from home as part of the COVID-19 restrictions in Melbourne from March until July 2020. I'm very grateful to my employer for enabling that to happen. I was pregnant at the time and even more focused on my health and safety in light of the little person who was getting ready to come into the world. On the downside, I found myself on a slippery slope to burnout as a mother of a toddler and with a heavy workload I was responsible for. Having to look after my son and work at the same time was no mean feat. I'm sure many parents around the world who found themselves home-schooling their children will have stories similar to mine they could share.

I have read articles that suggest drawing lines between our professional and personal lives is crucial from several points of view, not least of which is our mental health. But, holding the line can be difficult to achieve, even in the best of circumstances. This is where the question of boundaries rears its head. Research by the Harvard Business Review revealed that:

Workers often unintentionally make it hard for their supervisors, colleagues and employees to maintain boundaries. One way they do this is by sending work emails outside of office hours. In five studies involving more than 2000 working adults, it was found that senders of after-hours work emails underestimated how compelled the receivers felt to respond right away, even when the emails were not urgent.

I recall checking emails and responding to them all day long when I was working from home. This left me mentally drained and physically exhausted. I figured that everyone was going to be experiencing a heightened level of stress, panic and anxiety, so I had to play my part by being super-responsive. My sense was that the clinic business owners, in particular, would be working around the clock to make sure all of us would pull through as a collective, both from the financial and the project management perspective. I feel like some might have even needed to let go of some of their employees, but thankfully this was minimised by the Commonwealth Government subsidies that were made available in Australia.

The periods when we went into lockdown to manage the risks from Covid amplified the 'normal' pressures we were all under. Many schools were closed and day care was no longer an option. This placed additional burdens on working parents, especially those in low-income households. Even companies that already had employees working from home before Covid were likely to have trouble supporting those with the added challenge of maintaining their productivity in the presence of their families.

During that period, I pondered questions like: How might employees like me continue to compartmentalise their work and non-work lives? How can we 'leave our work at the door' if we don't actually go out any doors to get to work? What can employers, managers and co-workers do to help one another cope? And, most important of all, how do we stay *energised*?

Based on what I've learnt from the research and the wide range of other resources I've tapped into, I have three recommendations I want to share with you.

Maintain physical and social boundaries

In a classic paper, Blake Ashforth of the Arizona State University described the ways in which people demarcate the transition from work to non-work roles via 'boundary-crossing activities.' What he's referring to are things like putting on your work clothes and commuting between home and work. These are physical and social indicators that signal a transition from 'home you' to 'work you' has taken place.

I want to encourage you to try to maintain healthy boundaries when you are working remotely. In the short-term, working-from-home arrangements might feel like a welcome change because you don't have to catch an early train to work or get out of your tracksuit or, for that matter, your pyjamas. This might feel like a dream come true but getting dressed for work and leaving home to get there are boundary-crossing activities that actually do a great job of helping you to delineate your 'work life' and 'home life.' I would recommend you don't abandon things like getting dressed for work altogether. Perhaps you could replace your morning commute with a walk to a nearby park, or even just around your apartment, before you sit down to check your emails or whatever.

Maintain temporal boundaries as much as possible

Maintaining temporal boundaries is critical for *wellbeing* and *work engagement*. This is particularly true when so many of us are now facing the challenge of managing childcare or elder-care responsibilities during regular work hours. Thanks to the mobile devices that keep our work with us all the time, it's even challenging for employees without children or other family responsibilities.

Sticking to a 9-to-5 schedule may prove unrealistic but sticking as close as you can to it will help. Research confirms that people not only need to find work-time budgets that work for them, but they also need be conscious and respectful of the fact that others might work at different times than they do. For some, their 'no go' time might be when their child is having a nap. For others it might be when they are cooking dinner. People with or without children can create intentional work-time budgets by adding an 'out of office' reply on their email system during certain hours of the day so they can on focus on work that needs their undivided attention without interruption. A less extreme option might be to just let others know you might be slower than usual in responding to emails and, in doing so, managing expectations for others as well as yourself.

Keeping a sense of normality is key to everyone's wellbeing during this time of disruption. This calls for leaders to aid their employees in structuring, coordinating and managing the pace of work. It might entail holding regular virtual check-in meetings with employees or providing them with tools to create virtual coffee times or workspaces.

Focus on your most important work

Productivity can be a bit of a balancing act. The mundane tasks you can do with your eyes closed are important but setting aside time for the top-priority issues that take concentration can't be put in the too-hard basket because you're working from home. In other words, you need to allocate enough time and energy to do the things that fall outside the 'busy work' category.

I mention this here because it's been found that employees often feel compelled to project the appearance of productivity while they're working from home. This can result in focusing on tasks that are more immediate, instead of the less immediate but more important ones that take time and effort to complete. Research suggests this is a tendency that is counterproductive in the long run, even if it benefits productivity in the short-term.

Working all the time, even on your most important tasks, isn't the answer. According to some estimates, the average knowledge worker is only fully productive for about three hours every day. And for that to be the case (i.e. to get an average of three productive hours out of ourselves), the hours need to be free of interruptions and multitasking. Think about that for a moment. Even before Covid, employees found it difficult to carve out three continuous focused hours to get on with their core work. With work and family boundaries being removed, the potential for employees' time to be fragmented and their attention to be unfocused has never been more real.

Those who feel 'on' all the time are at a higher risk of burnout when working from home than they are when they leave home to go to a distinct workplace. In the long-term, trying to squeeze in work and email responses whenever we have a few minutes to spare (e.g. during the kids' nap time, on the weekend or by pausing a movie in the evening) is not only counterproductive but also detrimental to our wellbeing. What this all boils down to is that we all need to find new ways to carve out non-work time and mental space for ourselves.

I remember there was a sense that it wouldn't be for too long when we first went into lockdown. Indeed, in the scheme of things, it's fair to say that lockdowns have come and gone, but what we know now is that the 'new normal' seems to be here to stay. What this means is that, in many cases, working from home is going to be ongoing. Hybrid versions, where people might only go into the office one or two days a week, are proving to be particularly effective.

What we have to deal with now is the potential for a phase of post-Covid working-from-home burnout starting to rise to the surface. I see many working parents around me feeling exhausted and burnt out from the stress of the first eighteen months of Covid. Australians from the state of Victoria went through several severe lockdown periods between the time I started writing this book and when I finished it. My overall observation of the state of play is that most of us have built our resilience and strength with our heads held high. There is a kind of unspoken language when Victorians come together and talk about how we survived the pandemic. My sense is that, for the most part, we are now kinder and more compassionate towards one another.

Secret Ingredient Nine: Alignment
Choosing alignment over overwhelm

I used to regularly get sucked into the negative roadblocks and dramas in my life. A classic example of this was when I heaped blame on the person who was driving the car that hit me and rendered me a paraplegic. It may seem fair enough for me to feel aggrieved under the circumstances, but the point is that adopting that attitude caused me a lot of suffering.

Before, I had the driver who hit me to deflect blame from myself because, maybe, I wasn't doing everything I could have been doing to live life on my own terms. I blamed the healthcare system in general and the hospital I was working at, in particular. The grudge I held there was about being overworked and under-supported as a junior doctor. Sure, I was working exceptionally long, unpaid hours and no one cared, but did I ever speak up about it? No.

I even blamed the pandemic for everything that went wrong for me last year. Then the penny dropped and literally everything changed for me. I don't want you to take this the wrong way but I'm grateful to Covid because it put me in a place where I was open to learning the lesson that helped me shift my overwhelm into alignment. What I know now that I didn't know then, is that most people are overwhelmed because they don't understand how the Law of Vibration works. I live a life of high vibration every day now and because of that I feel less overwhelmed and, correspondingly, full of energy, motivation and inspiration.

The concept is simple. The key to wellbeing is to tap into the powerful force called the Law of Vibration. This is the real power source behind manifesting your desires. If you're like most people I know, you might think the game-changer is the Law of Attraction. I hear that a lot because of the hangover effect of the way it was popularised through the movie and the movement around *The Secret* by Rhonda Byrne which came out in 2006. Let's see what you think when you finish reading this chapter.

The possibilities are endless

The Law of Vibration states that anything that exists in our universe, whether visible or not, can be quantified as a frequency or an energetic pattern. All things carry their own unique vibration, from teeny tiny atoms – rainbows, light, stardust, dust on butterfly wings and happy thoughts – to more dense matter like rocks, thousand-year-old trees, dirt, bones, diamonds and metal.

It's a beautiful thing. As I choose happy feelings, more happy feelings will be drawn into vibrational harmony with the frequency I am living in. I've found that if I am constantly cranky and upset, then I will be attracting more of the same energy into my life. The Law of Vibration works like a big mirror. I create my vibrational set point, buzz that frequency out into the ether and whatever my dominant energetic patterns are will be drawn to me in the form of things, people and experiences that are in alignment with my vibration set point.

It looks like this: *Thoughts + Feelings + Actions + Intention = YOUR VIBRATION*

Your vibration then aligns with the order you are placing with God.

Then it looks like this: *ALIGNMENT = GOD'S ABILITY TO DELIVER*

To summarise:

- By consciously sculpting your energy (your vibration) you *activate* the Law of Vibration. You can then work with it to deliberately seek out ways to optimise your energy and clear the way for the alignment process to work its magic
- By aligning with your desires, and trusting they have already manifested on the etheric plane, you release any resistance and God can deliver your goodies because you have created a space for them to exist in.

Now, let's talk about the alignment process itself. I want you to really get a handle on this because it is the process you can use to activate the Law of Attraction in your life.

Here is what happens:

You set your intention (wish on a shooting star, daydream, map out your desires – whatever works for you). Then what you have wished for is officially 'out there.' The stage has been set and you can wonder how God will deliver your wishes. Meanwhile, there are a few key elements that people usually miss when they experiment with the manifesting process. One of them is knowing how to align your energy with your desires.

You see, being brilliant at dreaming up wonderful things to manifest in your life is the easy part. The tricky part is to align yourself with the things, the people and the experiences you want to attract. This is the key to unlocking the holding space for the goodies you are manifesting. The amazing thing is that over ninety per cent of the manifesting process has been completed by the time you get your vibration activated. This means the vibrational element of your wishes have already occurred in the non-physical realm. Your primary focus is to align yourself with your desires so they can appear in your physical reality.

I know I've already given you a lot to take in and I've probably massively challenged the left side of your brain but here's something else I really want you to absorb:

Everything happens in the etheric realm first.

Our physical realm is a mere echo of what happens in the etheric realm. Our task is to simply play catch-up and unlock the desires from the energetic holding space they're in so they can manifest in the 'real' world. In other words, all you need to do is close the gap between intention and manifestation.

Doing this is simple – act and feel as if your objects of desire have already appeared. In doing so, you will bridge the gap between the non-physical and the physical realms. This is not a new phenomenon. Manifestation exists in the Bible: *Ask, and it will be given to you; seek, and you will find; knock, and it will be opened to you. Matthew 7:7.*

Here is the roadmap to activate the Law of Attraction, using the process of alignment in four simple steps.

Step 1: Set your intentions from a space of clarity.

Step 2: Raise your vibration and feel good.

Step 3: Use the alignment process to act as if you have already manifested your desires. This draws them so much closer to you as you continue to raise your vibration.

Step 4: Trust, surrender, meditate and distract yourself because a watched pot never boils. Trust that God has your back and will deliver your intention in His timing.

If you are a power manifester, then life is in flow and you are always in a state of being happy with reality, no matter what shows up. Living in this state will imbue you with a wonderful sense of inner calm and peace.

In my role as a mentor and coach for doctors, I ask my clients to get clear about what they want. This gives them something tangible to aim for. The problem is that most people think that *goal-setting* is the answer – but goals can be hollow if they are not built on a strong foundation. How many times have you achieved a long sought-after goal, only to find it's not as satisfying as you thought it would be?

On the other hand, when meaningful goals are built on the foundation of purpose, values and mission, satisfaction is all but guaranteed.

The following questions will help you uncover your own purpose, values and mission:
- What is my life about?
- What do I value?
- What do I treasure?
- What is really important?
- What do I do in my life that is worthwhile?
- How do I want to be remembered?

As far as I'm concerned, being a conscious creator is the only way to go. I say that because when you are actively taking charge of your reality, you can master your fate. You can relax in the knowledge that, no matter what happens, you will be okay because you have all the tools you need in your spiritual toolbox. As long as your goals are set on the firm foundations of life – purpose, values and mission – you will be able to overcome anything and rise above it all.

Secret Ingredient Ten: Boldness
Choosing boldness over shame

Shame is the intensely painful feeling or experience of believing we are flawed and therefore unworthy of love, belonging and connection. According to Brené Brown, shame is the 'never good enough' emotion. It can stalk us over time, or completely ambush us in a second. Either way, its power is in making us feel we are not worthy of connection or belonging.

Before I dissect shame for you here, I want to walk you through the relevant parts of my backstory.

As you know, the accident that resulted in a serious injury to my spinal cord was a physically and emotionally traumatic event that changed my life forever. It might surprise you to know that the physical pain was nothing compared to the emotional suffering I endured for years. Knowing what I know now, it's clear to me that the emotional pain was, in large part, due to shame. In the first few years after my injury, I felt ashamed to the point of being mortified about my image as a person in a wheelchair. In fact, I was both ashamed and embarrassed. The difference between these emotions is that being ashamed relates to the way we think about ourselves and being embarrassed is about how we feel about what we think others think of us. I know what it's like to feel the sting of both of these emotions. There is no pun intended when I say I was crippled by the fear of people staring at me and judging me.

I had to use my wheelchair at work so I could conserve my energy for looking after my patients. I felt both shame and embarrassment when, all of a sudden, the senior doctors I'd worked with before my injury started to doubt my ability to do my job. The way they treated me, as a disabled person, made me feel useless and incompetent. You can imagine how effectively that environment compounded the negative self-talk I was perfectly capable of generating myself. The last thing I needed was people, who should respect me for my skill and diligence, heaping their unconscious bias on me. Needless to say, that seriously degraded my confidence and sense of self-worth. The only thing that stopped me from breaking down completely was the way in which my patients supported me and connected with me at an even deeper level than they did before the accident. It was as if I had become 'one of them' because I 'got where they were coming from.'

I struggled big-time with the shame and negative self-talk I had to handle over the years between the accident and my awakening through self-compassion. I used to be afraid to talk about shame. The paradox was that the less I talked about it, the more control it had over my life. Shame is the fear of disconnection. As I mentioned previously, we are physically, emotionally, cognitively and spiritually hardwired for connection, love and belonging. These things are core human needs. They give purpose and meaning to our lives. Shame is the fear of being unworthy of connection because of something we have done or failed to do, an ideal we have not lived up to or a goal we have not accomplished. Each time I achieved something, there was a little bully with a very loud voice in my head who would tell me, "You are never going to be good enough because you are not normal and able-bodied anymore." The bully also asked, "Who do you think you are? You will always be a nobody. You are in a wheelchair now and you are worthless."

Retreating into my shell became my modus operandi in the years before I found self-compassion because it felt like the easiest way to stay safe in the midst of my shame-fuelled self-talk that I couldn't seem to stamp out. What I couldn't see when I was in the depths of despair was that when I put my armour on and made myself small, things tended to break and I felt like I was suffocating.

The following dot points list some of the ways shame played out for me back in the day. As you read them, I'd like you to be thinking about how shame is playing out in your own life right now.

- Shame is trying to hide my spinal cord injury.
- Shame is my boss calling me incompetent in front of my colleagues and my patients.
- Shame is feeling proud of a project I've just completed, then being told it was not delivered to the standard my boss expected.
- Shame is failing my first long case examination in 2017.
- Shame is getting bullied at work in 2005 when I was an intern and being too afraid to say anything because the bully was the head of the department and a doctor who everyone loved.
- Shame is noticing that things changed when I returned to part-time work in 2012, and not being able to see how and where I could contribute. The fear of being irrelevant was a huge shame trigger when I went back to work.
- Shame is when the ward round had to slow down because I couldn't move fast without my wheelchair but I was too ashamed to use it.

Current neuroscience research shows the feelings of rejection that shame generates are very real and that getting out from under shame is not easy. Talking about the emotional pain generated by shame is even more difficult than talking about physical pain. In fact, shame derives its power from being unspoken. That's why a lot of people can't even say the word 'shame' without being triggered.

Research confirms that shame shows up in many ways at work. It can show up as:
- perfectionism
- favouritism
- gossiping
- back-channelling
- worth being totally tied to productivity
- harassment
- discrimination
- power over
- bullying
- blaming
- teasing
- cover-ups
- unconscious bias.

These are the kinds of behavioural cues that indicate shame has permeated a culture. Sadly, in medicine, shame has more than just permeated the culture – it has become an outright management tool. The cold hard truth of it is that people in medical leadership roles regularly bully others. They criticise subordinates in front of colleagues and deliver public reprimands or set up reward systems that intentionally embarrass, shame and humiliate the people they are targeting.

After going through what I've been through and watching others suffer within a broken system just like I have, I'm committed to working for change. What we need when it comes to enabling people to talk about shame is a space where they feel safe. That is to say, things need to be set up in the right way because there are powerful conversations to be had if the conditions are right. Giving people permission to talk about shame is liberating. It shines a light in a dark corner that makes it impossible for people to thrive. It's a wonderful thing to watch people realise they are not alone and they are not powerless. Sharing our stories enables connection and builds trust. It literally takes the power out of shame.

Brené Brown talks about shame resilience. This is the ability to turn up authenticity, even when we experience shame. It enables us to move through the experience we're being triggered by without sacrificing our values and to come out on the other side with more courage, compassion and connection than we had going into it. Ultimately, shame resilience is about moving from shame to empathy. Among other things, empathy is the antidote to shame.

I'm going to take this discussion up another notch now and fill you in on the fact that moving forward with boldness and really owning who you are without apology will shift you even faster into self-compassion.

Chris Germer, the author of several books on the topic of self-compassion, taught me to see the power of looking at shame through the eyes of self-compassion. You'll recall reading the chapter about choosing self-compassion over self-judgement earlier. Self-compassion is the opposite of shame. If you take nothing else out of reading this book, I want you to feel empowered to choose self-kindness instead of self-criticism; common humanity instead of isolation; and mindfulness instead of rumination.

Consider how different it feels to think about shame when we look at it as an innocent emotion that arises from the universal wish to be loved. It makes sense, doesn't it? The next step is to give ourselves the compassion we so desperately need and deserve. The world looks like a very different place when we look at it through the prism of self-compassion rather than self-criticism. I feel like Albert Einstein really nailed it when he said, "The most important decision we make every day is whether we live in a hostile world or not."

I was incredibly grateful to have had the opportunity to join a virtual workshop on *Mindful Self-Compassion,* run by Chris Germer in early March 2021. This training took a fresh, non-pathological look at shame through the eyes of compassion. I don't know about you, but I've done a lot of workshops and training that have felt pretty ground breaking when I'm doing them, but have had very little impact on me in the long run. This was not one of those. I was able to actually integrate the tools Chris shared and actually go out into the real world and use the contemplative practices I had learnt back at the hospital where I was working. What I found particularly helpful was being able to deconstruct the causes of shame, including the discrimination and social oppression that I saw playing out around me every day. This was especially relevant in the context of understanding the nature of the unconscious bias I was subjected to when I returned to work after my injury. I'm actually grateful for everything I've been through – I am only living the incredibly satisfying and purposeful life I'm living now because of the struggles I've been through.

Secret Ingredient Eleven: Love
The bridge of unconditional love

The Battle of Evermore began for me on the 23rd of March 2021. *The Battle of Evermore* is a song sung by Led Zeppelin and is commonly believed to be based on events in the final volume of J.R.R. Tolkien's *The Lord of The Rings*: *The Return of the King*.

In the months prior to that, I was struggling in a big way with balancing my medical work, my coaching business and motherhood. I was ignoring the signs of burnout and operating on the edge of exhaustion every day. I felt overworked and stressed and I was starting to feel invisible, isolated and unsupported. The entrepreneur world I'd dipped my toe into is such a noisy place, full of extroverts and attention-seekers. Among other things, I was falling into the trap of buying-in to the marketing hype around business strategies that were declared to always work. As it turns out, they usually don't. I was spending a lot of money and feeling like I was getting nowhere. It all got to be too much for me and I got to the point where it felt like I'd slipped right back to where I was when I fell headlong into burnout in 2018.

Being a medical entrepreneur was an isolating and lonely space to be in. I felt as if no one got me. The lack of support made me feel dissatisfied, frustrated, jaded and maybe even angry.

That wasn't the only problem, though. I actually started to lose heart in all aspects of my work and I was only managing to get through each day by simply working on autopilot. The way I was feeling was impacting my life beyond work as well. In fact, I was starting to lose my sense of self and confusing my identities as 'a doctor' and 'an entrepreneur.' Basically, I felt disconnected from myself and my passion.

I started feeling quite unwell with what felt like a viral illness in the couple of days prior to the 23rd of March. I had a fever, sweats and rigors and my joints were aching. Yet, in spite of feeling terrible, I pushed through with neither my medical work nor my creative business suffering. I was relying on the cashflow from my medical work to feed into getting my creative business off the ground. I was spending way too much money on things that weren't generating revenue and, emotionally, I was sinking into despair while my body was falling apart.

On that fateful day in March, I woke up with intense pain in my right leg. The leg itself was turning red and swelling up like a balloon. I immediately put my 'doctor hat' on and diagnosed myself with cellulitis. I made an appointment with my GP who told me to get myself down to the Emergency Department at the hospital straight away. I didn't need an ambulance but the tone in my doctor's voice made it very clear that things were serious. Again, I got to see what it's like on the other side of the healthcare system.

I have to say I was seriously disappointed with the poor level of care I received in the Emergency Department. There was a notable lack of compassion from everyone – from the triage nurse to the junior doctors and other nurses in the Emergency Department. Fortunately, Dr Steve saved the day. He was the one who attended to me while I was waiting in the clinic of the Emergency Department. On a side note, I had been wrongly triaged by the triage nurse in the first place. I should have actually been cared for at the Short Stay Unit. Nevertheless, Dr Steve immediately diagnosed me with cellulitis and decided to admit me as an inpatient so I could receive intravenous (IV) antibiotics for a couple of days. He started asking me about my family and, once he knew I was a doctor, about my medical work. It turned out that, like me, he had two kids and was interested in how I managed to balance having a family and working in medicine. His youngest was only seven weeks old. What struck me about Dr Steve, in contrast to the other medical staff I had dealt with before he arrived, was that he spoke to me in a polite and friendly manner that would make anyone feel at ease.

Soon after I arrived in the Short Stay Unit, I decided to have myself transferred to a private hospital to receive the kind of medical treatment I needed. I'm not a snob about these kinds of things but I waited for seventeen hours in the Short Stay Unit as my body was starting to deteriorate, with signs of septic shock becoming apparent. I was appalled by the fact the medical and nursing staff barely attended to my care at all and critically failed to institute the medical treatment I needed as a person whose body was going into the dangerous state of septic shock.

It was actually the patient transport team that arrived to take me to the private hospital who flagged that I was in septic shock. During those moments where I was starting to lose consciousness, my mind drifted to my children, my husband, my medical career and my creative business. I was asking myself if I'd achieved my goals and dreams. Had I left my children the legacy of teaching them to follow their heart's desire and pursue their dreams? I started to panic about not having done those things yet and I felt myself sinking into despair. I started blaming myself for ignoring the symptoms of the infection that landed me in hospital.

I don't know how it happened but just as I was recognising I wasn't in a position to leave my children the kind of legacy I want to leave them, something clicked and I started to use the C.I.A. formula I had learnt. C.I.A. stands for compassion, intuition and attitude. This is the methodology I now teach my coaching clients.

With compassion, I acknowledged I was suffering from pain and illness. *This was the mindful awareness component of compassion* playing out in the real world. I felt connected to the other patients in the Short Stay Unit who were there for their own various illnesses. We were all suffering together. *This was the common humanity pillar of self-compassion.* I began to accept that it is what it is – I had cellulitis that I needed medical treatment for. It was not my fault. *This was the self-acceptance pillar of self-compassion.*

Then I started to use my intuition. I started to tune in to the energy of the Short Stay Unit and I meditated intuitively. I saw the greatness in the people around me and the greatness in myself. I saw my infection for what it was, neither good nor bad. I saw the medical and nursing staff for who they were, neither good nor bad. I started to see my egoic structure for what it was, and I also saw I had a choice to give the power to my higher self. And that is what I did.

My attitude completely changed after I tapped into compassion, followed by intuition. I was more relaxed and I was open to receive. At that point, I started to radically awaken, and I vowed to carry on creating the legacy of the work I was doing as a physician, speaker, author, mentor and coach for other doctors. I *chose* for my vitals to be stable enough for me to be able to make it to the private hospital to continue my medical care, with the end result of getting better. My clinical condition stabilised in a few hours. When the patient transport team came to collect me for the second time, I was happy to see them. Their presence meant I was one step closer to receiving the medical treatment I deserved in the private hospital. I wasn't disappointed. I did indeed receive the best medical care available in the private hospital and was discharged to go home under Hospital in the Home (HITH) conditions a few days after I had been admitted. The doctors and nurses looked after me impeccably. After a further three and a half weeks on intravenous antibiotics, I was discharged from HITH.

As I write this chapter, a week after being discharged from HITH, I am now back on duty with my medical work and I'm slowly getting back to my coaching business. As I reflected on my most recent hospital experience, I realised the episode with cellulitis had a silver lining. It forced me to have all the rest I so desperately needed. I got to spend quality time with my son, Joseph, who was on school holidays at the time, and my eight-month-old daughter, Jacqueline. I also got to read a bunch of great self-help and personal development books that I hadn't found time to read previously. I nourished myself with rest, quality relationships and learning to love myself unconditionally once again.

Things happen for a reason. The Battle of Evermore happened; I survived it and am ready to be the awakened physician and medical entrepreneur who carries on doing good work to positively impact the lives of those around me. I have been reborn. Radically awakened. Ready to make the next quantum leap.

Secret Ingredient Twelve: Freedom
Choosing freedom over burnout

In 2020 when the world was being tipped upside down by Covid-19, I finally got to the point where I wanted to rediscover the passion in my work, restore my mental and emotional wellbeing, and reconnect with my family, my inner self, and my identity. I had lost sight of who I was beyond being a physician. In the process of reconnecting with the important facets of my life and myself, I found a renewed sense of purpose and clarity in my mission to help doctors around the world to lead the heart-centred life they truly deserve.

This period of honing my focus started to really take shape when I discovered a number of powerful self-compassion and personal development tools that helped me get to a place where I was thriving at home and at work. Through these tools I also learnt how to take ownership of my thoughts and gain a whole new perspective on life.

Not only was I sick and tired of living with fatigue and overwhelm, but I was determined to chart a course of change that others who were coming behind me could follow.

I had a fire in my belly because I've seen way too many of my talented medical colleagues burn out as I had done myself (not once, but twice). So I worked on this problem as diligently as I've ever worked on anything in my life, and I figured out how I could help my peers discover the heart-based tools that had helped me get out of the hole I was in.

I've seen burnout from both sides, and I'm passionate about arming my colleagues with powerful tools they can use to rediscover their self-worth and lead the kind of heart-centred life I've been able to establish for myself. I want to help them find that spark of joy and creativity outside the world of medicine like I have, and access the freedom to do whatever they want. In other words, I want to put the power back in their hands.

Quietly shaking up the status quo in this way led me to develop a leadership program and become a leadership coach for doctors. My mission in life is now all about opening the options up for highly qualified people who are being worn out by an under-resourced system that is bleeding them dry.

In this chapter, I will be introducing you to a powerful transformational tool I've developed called *The Five Keys to Freedom*. This is the foundation of the coaching program I use to help my clients transform their lives. My global personal brand - *The Heart-Centred Doctor,* is driven by the fact that we need more heart-centred people in medicine who can go the distance with as much passion for their work as they had when they first started.

After overcoming adversity both inside and outside the medical profession, I have finally found my WHY. This is what I want for you.

The Five Keys to Freedom

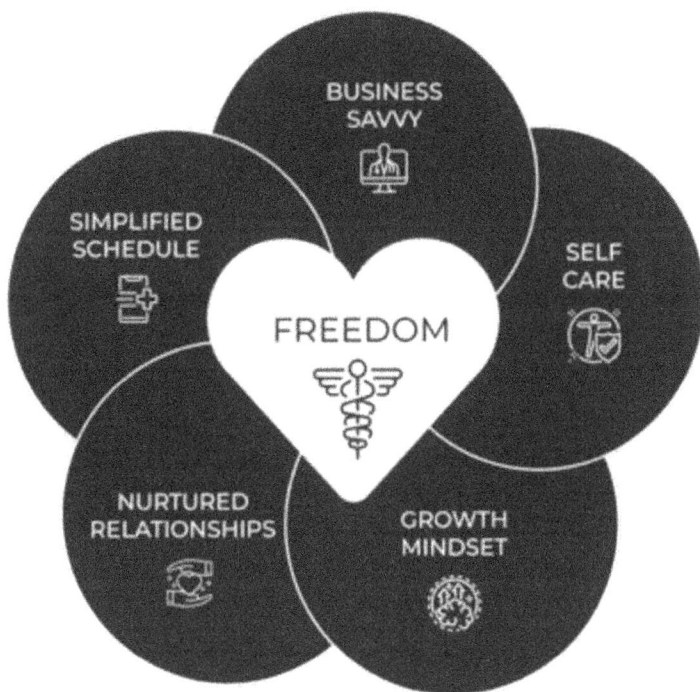

The five keys to getting to a place of **FREEDOM** that you might not even be able to imagine right now, include practicing self-care; having a growth mindset; nurturing our relationships; simplifying our schedules; and developing what I call our 'business savvy'. We're going to look at each of these in turn now.

1. Self-Care

As a female physician who is a mum, a wife, and an entrepreneur, I used to regularly catch myself filling the cups of others before filling my own. From a cultural standpoint, this was expected. The only problem was that when I was busy serving my family, communities, patients, and the teams of medical professionals I worked with from a half-filled cup, low hanging emotions tended to rise to the surface and compromise my effectiveness in all areas of my life. The kind of emotions I'm talking about here are resentment, anxiety, stress, and worry. These were bubbling to the surface when I was continually stretching myself too thin back in the days before I worked out how to restore my life to a place of balance and fulfillment.

It wasn't until I started taking my immediate and future wellbeing seriously and regularly tapping into a well of compassion for myself that I realised filling my cup needed to be a non-negotiable priority. I'm very grateful that I got to see the importance of setting myself up with a better mindset than the one that spiralled out of control and ended in burnout. Basically, I needed a new way of thinking that put self-care front and centre when it came to the way I ran my life. One thing I learnt pretty quickly was that far from being selfish, self-care is about taking responsibility for my own wellbeing so that I'm able to lead the way for others who want to follow my example and choose freedom over burnout for themselves.

The fundamentals of self-care are not complicated, but because of the complicated lives so many of us live, it can seem as if they are. Basically, it's about making sure we get enough sleep, keep our bodies well-nourished in terms of the food we eat, and keep our hearts full in terms of the relationships we have in the home, the workplace, and the other circles we move in. This is important, so I'm going to spell out exactly what I mean by breaking this down into six key components. They are the physical, mental, emotional, spiritual, relationship, and workplace aspects of self-care that we need to master to develop an environment where we can thrive.

Here's what the physical aspect of self-care includes:
- eating regular healthy meals
- drinking plenty of water
- taking time off when you're sick
- enjoying regular exercise

- thinking positively about your body
- getting massages
- getting enough sleep
- wearing clothes that you like
- getting regular medical care
- eating food that you love without guilt
- getting outside each day.

Here's what the mental aspect of self-care includes:
- making time for self-reflection
- taking day trips or mini-vacations
- having an outlet for creativity
- taking time away from the internet and technology
- practicing stress reduction
- learning new things
- reading things unrelated to work
- saying no to extra responsibilities
- being okay to leave work at work.

Here's what the emotional aspect of self-care includes:
- spending time with friends
- finding things that make you laugh
- loving yourself
- expressing your frustration in healthy ways
- allowing yourself to cry
- giving yourself affirmation and praise
- comforting yourself in healthy ways.

Here's what the spiritual aspect of self-care includes:
- having a spiritual connection or community
- connecting to what is meaningful to you
- praying, meditating, or engaging in other practices regularly
- practicing gratitude
- contributing to causes that you believe in

- reading inspirational materials
- spending time in nature
- paying attention to everyday beauty
- having a sense of meaning and purpose.

Here's what self-care in the area of relationships includes:
- having regular dates with your partner
- calling or visiting your relatives
- making time to be with friends
- spending time with animals
- keeping in contact with friends who are far away
- sharing hopes and fears with someone you trust
- asking for help when you need it
- allowing others to do things for you.

Here's what self-care in the workplace includes:
- taking time to chat with co-workers
- identifying and taking on tasks that are exciting
- arranging your workspace so that it's comfortable
- taking a break and, if possible, getting out into the sunshine during the day
- negotiating and advocating for your needs
- setting limits with your boss and peers.

Ultimately self-care is about striking a balance between work and free time; between time with the family and time alone; and between looking forward to things in the future and staying present.

2. Growth Mindset

This section on mindset is about skilling you up to work with your mind so that it empowers you to develop and grow as long as your heart is beating, rather than believing your options are limited by the talents you were born with.

The chapters you've already read have been focused on introducing you to heart-based tools that will help you to be more present. What we're addressing here is the fact that even if we master the art of being present, our results are still likely to be a projection of our past thoughts and programming. The good news is that we can reorient our projections and beliefs because they are determined by the extent to which we operate from a fixed or a growth mindset.

I want to tease this out a bit more by taking a look at how our mind works. Don't worry, I'm going to keep this as simple as pointing out that when an event happens, it generates a thought. Then that thought generates other thoughts that our mind gets busy constructing meanings around, while at the same time our emotions are being triggered. Because all of this happens within a millisecond, it might sound strange to say that we are making choices all along this chain of causation. But it's true, and what we choose to think will determine the emotion we experience, and in turn that will determine the action we take. What this means is that the journey we take from having a thought to having an outcome looks a bit like this.

Event ⇨ Thought ⇨ Multiple thinking ⇨ Emotions ⇨ Action ⇨ Outcome

It's important to note that our brain is hardwired to take the path of least resistance, so to save energy it automates our responses as much as possible. This can cause problems because it might result in our staying stuck in unresourceful states playing out unhelpful patterns over and over again. So, what we're going to look at now is a way to approach life with empowered thinking rather than settling for the path of least resistance that ensures the status quo is maintained.

Empowered thinking

At the most basic level, empowered thinking comes down to exercising choice and opening your awareness. You can change the way you think by applying the two points below.

1. Gaining awareness. This starts by observing your thoughts and your thinking patterns.
2. Once you've got a handle on the way you think, it's about choosing a more empowered way of thinking. To do that, you can simply ask yourself what's a more empowering thing I could be thinking to increase my chances of getting the outcome I want.

You might be thinking there must be more to it than that. Well, actually there is. It's about repeating these two points again and again so that you build new neural pathways in your brain. This is the key to establishing empowered thinking as your default state.

Socratic questioning

Another way to transform the way you think is called Socratic questioning. This is a disciplined questioning process that will enable you to establish what is true and what is not. It's also effective at revealing any underlying assumptions that might be at play in the back of your mind. Socratic questioning is based on the four principles below:

1. Challenge any unresourceful thoughts that come to mind by asking yourself if that is true.
2. Consider alternative perspectives by asking yourself if that is the best way for you to approach the situation at hand.
3. Try a different way of thinking by asking yourself what a more empowered way to be thinking about this would look like.

4. Embody empowered thinking by asking yourself if you could try the more empowered way of thinking you identified above to create consistent progress in the direction of your desired outcome.

Applying these four simple strategies will not only help you step into an empowered thinking cycle in the short term. It will also change the way you think in the long term as well.

Note: Just because these strategies are simple doesn't mean it's easy to make them your default position. So don't beat yourself up if you don't 'remember' to apply these strategies every time the opportunity arises. The mind can be tricky, and one thing it's very good at is maintaining the status quo. In other words, don't lose heart if you look back on a situation that didn't turn out how you would have liked because you were undermined by unempowering thoughts. Just take note of what happened and use it as an opportunity to run through the alternative version of events using the four empowering steps above. This time I want you to actually write your answers down. I've put some examples from my own experience in here so that you can get the hang of how this works.

1. The unresourceful thought that came to mind when .... happened was ....

- When I asked myself if it was true, the answer that came to mind was - only if I believe it to be true, and don't do the work to change the way I look at things.

2. This is what happened when I considered other ways I could be thinking about ....

- I realised that things were never going to change if I didn't push through my old patterns and try something new, and

I reminded myself that saying I was going to start doing this tomorrow wasn't going to cut it anymore because if I listed everything I said I was going to start doing tomorrow yesterday, there would be at least four things on that list that hadn't been done yet.

3. When I asked myself what a more empowered way of thinking would look like, I came up with this.
- This is all about being open to change and showing myself compassion about maybe not always getting it right, and having an unwavering determination to do the work to get to where I want to be. I'm sick of being stuck and I'm going to do whatever it takes to change.

4. When I asked myself whether I could try a more empowered way of thinking to create consistent progress in the direction of my desired outcome, this is what came to mind.

- This is all about not stopping short and failing to take action like I've done so many times in the past. It's about being prepared to go the distance and follow through by taking empowered action.

Why something as apparently simple as this works is because if we are prepared to do the work to grow some new neural networks and start consistently thinking differently, we will be aligning the five elements that create our reality to deliver positive results.

These five elements are:
- The words we speak
- The thoughts we think
- The beliefs we hold
- The emotions we feel
- The actions we take.

After a fair bit of trial and error and plenty of research, I devised a process based on the **L.I.C.A. Method**. This process involves Listening, Identifying, and Choosing to Act. I use it to skill my clients up to work on the words they speak and the thoughts they think to change the results they are getting. This is how this four-step process plays out.

Step 1: Listen

I help my clients hone their awareness on the things they say to themselves so that they can see how they are literally talking themselves out of making the changes they need to make. Here's what I ask my clients to help them to lean in and listen to the words the voice in their head is using:

1. What are some of the thoughts that crossed your mind when …. happened?
2. Now list the words your mind used to represent these thoughts.

Words matter because they don't just express our thoughts, they also shape them in a way that is meaningful to us.

Step 2: Identify

What we need to do next is identify whether these thoughts (and the words that we associate with them) represent a growth or a fixed mindset. The questions below can help us here.

- Do you think the thoughts you identified above are true? Can you absolutely know they are true?
- Can you give me an example to support the decision you made to think they are true?
- What mindset do you think you were operating from here?

NB: If you're not sure, come back to this question when you've read the material below on the characteristics of fixed and growth mindsets.

Fixed vs growth mindset

Dr. Carol Dweck is a researcher at Stanford University and the author of *Mindset: The New Psychology of Success.* She talks about two types of mindsets: Growth and Fixed.

Basically, we have a fixed mindset if we believe the qualities we are born with are carved in stone. In other words, the talents and personality traits we are born with are the ones we have for the rest of our life. This means we have a fixed amount of intelligence, a cheery (or not) personality, and a high moral character (or not). A consequence of the belief that these kinds of things are fixed is that we are going to be noticing things that prove we are right and filtering out those that would prove we are wrong. A corollary of having a fixed mindset is that we will believe that there is no point in even trying things that we don't think we're any good at because we will only fail.

Whereas if we have a growth mindset, we believe the qualities we are born with are only a starting point, and we can learn and grow for as long as we live. Obviously, this is a much more empowering way to think with an attitude driven by the belief that our development in any area of our life can be cultivated as long as we put in the effort to learn and acquire new skills. This perspective leads us to be inquisitive, curious, interested in what others say, and open to exploring new ways of approaching life.

I believe the reality is not quite as clean-cut as having one mindset at the exclusion of the other, but rather, that we might approach some areas of our life with a fixed mindset and others with a growth mindset, and we can even lapse into a growth mindset from time to time if we're predominantly a person who operates through a fixed mindset and vice versa. The point is that once you're aware of what's going on, you can deliberately take your tendency toward a growth mindset from one area of your life and transfer it to another.

So let's take a closer look at which words represent lack and tend to dominate the language of people with a fixed mindset, and which ones represent opportunity and are more likely to come out of the mouths of people with a growth mindset.

Words of Lack include:
- Should
- Can't
- Ought to
- Have to
- The problem is
- But
- It's not fair
- I hate this
- I don't know
- This will never work.

Words of abundance include:
- I want to
- I choose to
- I get to
- I can
- And (rather than 'but')
- The solution might be
- Sometimes.

Here are some examples to help you get your head around this.

What a fixed mindset sounds like	What a growth mindset sounds like
I can't do that.	I'm not sure I can do it now, but I think I can learn to do it with time and effort.
What if I fail? I'll be a failure!	Most successful people have had failures along the way. Failure is a part of life.
I'm talented when it comes to words, but I can't draw to save my life.	Even those with the greatest inherent talent need to work hard to succeed in their field. I'm prepared to give anything a go and put the effort in to developing my skill in anything that lights me up.
I'm no good at this kind of stuff. It's not my strong suit!	I can figure this out even if it takes me longer than people who are naturals when it comes to this stuff. Are there classes I can take, people I can ask for help, or any other resources I could tap into?

Freedom to choose

What a lot of people don't realise is that they are able to choose how they feel about a problem. In fact, getting a handle on the power of choice has played a massive role in the adversity I've been able to overcome myself, and the things I see my clients achieving once they get out of their own way.

Here are a couple of questions that will help you to develop a growth mindset that is based on the belief that you deserve to choose the way you think about what goes on in your life and the opportunities that are out there for you to seize:

- What if the opposite is true?
- What can I learn from this situation?
- How did this situation help me grow?

The importance of action

Taking the kind of action a person with a growth mindset would take is absolutely integral to our ability to live an empowered life. If you're not sure how that would look, you could start by asking yourself these powerful questions:

- What steps could I take to get closer to my idea of success?
- What do I need to believe to avoid all the thoughts that have stopped me from taking the steps I identified above?
- What will I say to myself if any of these thoughts emerge as I move through the steps I need to take to achieve my goals?
- How will I celebrate when I achieve each of the goals I set on my way to my idea of success?

As my mentor and transformational coach Michael Neil wrote in his book *The Inside-Out Revolution:*

Our experience of life is created from the inside out via the principles of Mind, Consciousness, and Thought. We're living in the feeling of our thinking, not the feeling of the world.

In *The Inside-Out Revolution,* Michael talks about the fact that the implications of a simple shift in understanding can be profound because once we realise that our experience of life is not being created by our circumstances, we can break free from the belief that we need to change the world in order to change the way we feel and the results we get. If you think about it, approaching life from this perspective has far-reaching implications. I say that because if our experience is not being created by other people, then we don't need to try to control their behaviour (or submit to their control) in order to feel happy, loved, and whole.

This goes further than our relationship with others. Perhaps more importantly, it has profound implications for our relationship with ourselves. And in the relative peace and quiet of no longer feeling like we have to change, control, or fear the world around or within us, we're able to tap into the innate inner world of silence, beauty, and wonder that we lost touch with somewhere along the way. As Michael says, the beauty of all of this is that we will fill up with the simple feeling of being alive and enjoy the 'aliveness' at the heart of who we really are. In this state we get to experience a depth of love and gratitude that is both the reward most of us seek, and the direct path to tapping in to more of it. From that place of peace and wellbeing, we're both more present in the world and more available to others. This is a great place to be because our brain seems to work better, our common sense emerges, and we are able to make inspired leaps in our work and personal life. In a nutshell - we absolutely thrive.

3. Nurtured Relationships

It's helpful to remember that relationships are living things. They need to be nurtured because if we're not prioritising the important people in our life by giving them the time and the energy they deserve, our relationship with them is likely to wither and potentially die. Relationships are important because they effect every other area of our life. Our success within the business/career side of our life comes down to the quality of our relationships with customers, colleagues, managers, suppliers, banks, etc. Even the internet opens us up to a range of relationships with other people. And then of course there's the question of our relationship with ourselves and how well we practice self-care and self-love. This matters because when you think about it, our physical health and our emotions are simply a reflection of the relationship we have with ourselves. We can take this even further and consider the extent to which our finances are not only a reflection of the relationships we have within our workplace and/or business, but also a reflection of our mindset.

There's a whole book I could write about the importance of having a positive mindset around money, but for now, I want you to just be thinking broadly about the importance of investing time and energy in developing a set of healthy beliefs around things as (apparently) disparate as spirituality and financial wellbeing.

The bottom line is that as leaders of our own lives, the most significant factor affecting our ability to change is the degree to which we accept that we get to choose our emotional state. This is important because doing the work to get into that state of 'knowing' and 'being' will change our behaviour, which in turn will change the physiology of our body, right down to the biochemistry of our cells.

This isn't just about recognising when we feel happy, angry, or sad. The kind of awareness I'm referring to here is about noticing all of our emotions, and then on the basis of understanding what's really going on (especially if we're in the middle of a drama of some kind), deliberately making conscious choices about whether we need to take action, or whether it's best to leave things alone.

As with the sensations we feel in our body, being mindful of our emotions creates practical awareness of the state we're in at any given time. Among other things, this will allow us to recognise when we're too close to the edge before we actually topple over it. Imagine shaking up a bottle of carbonated soda and watching the pressure mount. I want you to bring that image to mind because bottling up our emotions creates a similar kind of internal pressure that takes us right out of the part of our brain that's responsible for making informed decisions and bumps us into the prehistoric part of our brain where our instinct for fight or flight takes hold. Now don't get me wrong. The flight or fight response is an incredibly empowering state when we're being chased down the street by an axe-wielding murderer, but not so much when we're having a disagreement with our partner about who's turn it is to do the dishes.

The point I want to drive home here is that things like awareness and acceptance are powerful tools that will make it much easier for you to deal with challenging emotions and circumstances whenever they arise. Simply describing and labelling how we feel can decrease the hold our emotions have over us and bring us into a state where our prehistoric instincts aren't running the show. It's important to get a handle on this because there are moments in life that are hard, painful, scary, and difficult to live through. And these are the times when we're likely to feel anger, anxiety, grief, embarrassment, stress, remorse, or other unpleasant emotions. In trying times like these we instinctively look for ways to escape the pain by drowning it out or pushing it away somehow. We might even get involved in a mental struggle with the pain where in a sense, we're trying to mentally talk our way out of it. Or we might distract ourselves by being super busy all the time or drown it out with food or drink or something stronger. These strategies might give us a degree of respite in the short term, but in the long run they will only perpetuate the problem.

I want you to really take this on board because things like avoidance and denial ultimately increase our suffering and stop us from living a fully satisfying life. The thing I want you to be aware of is that we normally react to pain or discomfort in one of two ways. One of them is called 'blocking', and the other is 'drowning'.

In the case of blocking, we try to negate the discomfort we're feeling by pushing through it using the force of will. Or maybe we distract ourselves, or numb ourselves through self-medicating with food, alcohol or drugs. Unfortunately, this doesn't work because our emotions will come back even stronger as soon as we stop doing whatever we're doing to keep them at bay. This is especially problematic in cases where the discomfort is a sign that corrective action needs to be taken, because missing these signs could result in injury, disease or even death. And, of course, self-medicating has the potential to undermine our wellbeing with complex side-effects and even addiction which will take the negative effects of avoidance and denial to a whole other level.

On the other hand, we're likely to become overwhelmed by our problems in the case of drowning. It often feels as if we're being dragged under by the discomfort we're in, and as we become more and more incapacitated by a sense of hopelessness and powerlessness it literally feels as if we're being subsumed by the weight of our circumstances.

The fact that we might resort to blocking or drowning makes a lot of sense because in the process of growing up and moving from schools to workplaces, most of us are taught that to feel emotion is a sign of weakness. And to avoid feeling weak, we will do whatever we need to do to alleviate any painful emotions that might emerge. We often do this with the help of things like food, alcohol, and drugs. Or we might distract ourselves by staying busy or getting involved in dramas of one kind or other. It's bad enough that drowning and blocking do nothing to help us to solve our problems, but worse still, continuing to rely on these strategies to keep painful emotions at bay is likely to make things even worse than they were in the first place.

Basically, the challenges my coaching clients come to me for help with are the result of the interplay between their behaviours and their emotions. They often tell me they feel like giving up because they're plagued with an overarching sense of powerlessness, hopelessness and overwhelm. These are classic signs of drowning. Or they might complain that they're piling on the weight because they can't stop binging, or they feel guilty and ashamed, not to mention worried about the health consequences of the drugs they've been using to numb the frustration and rage building up inside of them. These people are using blocking strategies to get by.

How to handle challenging behaviour

What I help my clients see is that our behaviours are backed up by thinking patterns that we repeat over and over again. Unless we are conscious of what's going on, we will be stuck on autopilot and unable to work out what to do to get out of the rut we've found ourselves in.

For example, I had a client who told me she was a procrastinator, and that she was feeling really frustrated about never being able to make progress toward any of her goals. I asked her a number of questions that helped her see that sometimes she procrastinates because she is not intrinsically motivated, and other times it's because the task she is faced with is new to her or it requires more effort than she wants to put in. What she was able to identify when we teased this out is that she often gets stuck in a cycle of trying to simplify processes, and if that doesn't work, she just keeps going around in circles. This was an important piece of awareness for her because she got to see that this is the strategy that maintains her resistance to just getting down to doing the work she needs to do to achieve her goals. As we talked about this my client realised that telling herself that she is not intrinsically motivated, or that she needs to simplify the problem before she starts working on it is just a well-worn pattern that she'd been playing out in her mind for decades. So I invited her to think about where her thoughts were coming from. What I was trying to get to the bottom of was exactly what feelings trigger the thinking that triggers the behaviour that she calls procrastination. Once we got to the bottom of that she was able to untangle her identity with the label of procrastination. So procrastination is now a thing that she might catch herself doing from time to time, but it does not define who she is anymore.

For my clients (and for you if you're reading this book because your life isn't panning out the way you had planned), breaking free from patterns of thinking and behaviours that are stopping you from getting to where you want to be starts with identifying the thinking that precedes the behaviour that is sabotaging your efforts to achieve your goals. Once we can recognise the repetitive thinking that's playing out, we can challenge it and change the behaviour associated with it.

You could think of it like this:

Event ⇨ Thought ⇨ Multiple thinking ⇨ Emotions ⇨ Action ⇨ Outcomes

Most of the clients I work with come to me because they can't seem to change repetitive behaviours that are causing them problems. As a coach, I have to be mindful that not all of the behaviours my clients perceive as being 'bad' are actually bad for them. One thing I need to make sure of is whether the change they want to make is being motivated by what's intrinsically right for them, versus what the external world says they should be doing. I am not here to judge a client's behaviour, but rather help them identify whether something is serving them or not. If it's not, then I help them shift it.

How to handle challenging emotions

We're really honing in on the question of emotions now. Emotions happen as a consequence of the way we think about what happens to us. I make that point because it's our emotional state that inspires action. And if we choose a different way of thinking, our emotions will show up differently, and in turn the emotions we experience will inspire us to take different actions.

The thing is that we have to be able to move through our emotional states rapidly to evolve to a higher state of consciousness. And it's worth doing the work to move to a higher state of consciousness because that's the easiest (if not the only) place to take inspired action. Every action we take is a physical manifestation of an emotional response. So, success comes down to the extent to which we can manage our emotions so that we can manage our actions in a way that will get us the outcomes we want.

How to get into a more positive and inspired state

What I want to say here is that there is nothing wrong with experiencing the whole range of emotions. In fact, that's what life is all about. The key is to learn how to efficiently move through painful emotions to a more empowered state that serves you, rather than getting stuck in your painful emotions. It's important to note that some emotional states come from psychological challenges that I am not qualified to help with. For conditions like deep depression for example, I recommend you refer yourself to a licensed therapist.

Notwithstanding the disclaimer above, whatever state you're in at the moment, it's worth taking steps to empower yourself with tools to manage emotionally charged situations. I say that because it would be a rare person who goes through life without finding themselves in an emotionally challenging space from time to time.

I find the four steps below work really well in most cases.

1. Identify the emotional state you're in by asking yourself what emotion is coming up for you now.
2. Slow yourself down because you have to be calm before you can think clearly.
3. Rationalise the situation by disassociating yourself from the emotion so that you can make a decision about how to move forward with a clear head. Remember, your emotions are a response to your thinking and vice versa. So to manage your emotions, you have to be aware of your thoughts.
4. Take the state of a detached observer by seeing the situation like an outsider would see it (kind of like watching a movie). This perspective will allow you to consider all options including empathy and compassion

Among other things, once you've processed the emotion you identify you will be in a much better state to communicate with the other party in a case where someone else is involved.

In his book *Nonviolent Communication,* Marshall B. Rosenberg outlines a slightly different approach that I find really helpful. The touch points he identifies are –

1. Observation
2. Identify a feeling
3. Identify your need or desire
4. Formulate a request.

As well as processing emotions, this approach will also work if you want to get a handle on your self-talk. That might sound a bit weird, but I recommend that you give it a go. It could literally change your life. It's about formulating a request to the voice in your head that's good at talking you out of doing things you know you need to do to achieve the goals you set for yourself.

What we're aiming for here is a middle ground. It's that place where you're neither pushing difficult feelings or situations away, nor being subsumed by them. This middle ground involves learning how to 'feel' the sensations or emotions in your body without being swept away by them. You might find it hard to believe that this is even possible if you've never tried to do something like this before, but I promise you it is.

There are three ingredients that make this even more powerful and effective. They are:
• Compassion and non-judgment
• Empathy (not sympathy)
• Honesty.

This piece from Stephen Cope's book *Yoga and the Quest for the True Self* sums this up beautifully:

The path, from the very first step, is self-acceptance. The goal is self-acceptance. The fruit of this practice is self-love. Compassion for the self and compassion for others radiates naturally from every moment of practice. As we practice allowing and accepting, we open our hearts and embrace that part of ourselves, or that part of another, that has been pushed away. By cherishing, honouring, allowing all our energies, we move into that place inside that says "yes" to all experience. Yes! Through "yes" we have stepped into the plane of consciousness of the fully alive human being."

---

4. Simplified Schedule

On a more practical note, a lot of the stress doctors are under comes from the almost superhuman level of organization they need to apply in an environment that is chronically under-resourced. Notwithstanding the resourcing issues, their personal productivity and wellbeing is also compromised by things they can readily do something about. What I'm talking about here are things like:

- Interruptions
- Procrastination
- Not setting the right priorities
- Poor planning
- Failing to delegate
- Not setting or maintaining boundaries
- Lacking focus
- Not being prepared to say no
- Not allocating enough time for administration and self-care.

Hence, we need to simplify and conscientiously manage our schedules. It's that simple. This might involve reducing the number of clinics you're working in. Or it might be about getting out of the habit of refusing to stop doing things that take up energy but give you nothing in return. If you get nothing else out of reading this book, I want you to get the energy to simplify your schedule so that you can get everything you need to do finished without living under so much pressure that burnout is only one drama of some kind or other away. This is not about becoming superhuman. It's about being sensible and practicing a reasonable amount of self-care.

I've written this book because I see too many people in the medical profession going about their jobs as if they're in a sprint rather than a marathon. The appalling statistics around burnout and worse suggest that we can't keep rewarding people for operating this way. It is dangerous, unfair, and unsustainable.

I know this is true because I've experienced burnout myself, and I'm grateful to have found a number of tools that have enabled me to take inspired action to overcome the time management and other challenges that led me down the dark path to burnout not so long ago. Two tools that I want to share with you here are the P.G.P.T. Formula and the F.A.S.T Formula. Applying these tools have made a big difference in my life. And several clients have reported that they've helped them to get some balance back in their lives. These results were possible because being more organised at work has elevated their productivity and made time for them to regenerate both their personal and professional life.

The P.G.P.T Formula

This four-part formula combines the **P**omodoro Technique with the idea of **G**athering all of the required information into one place, and applying **P**areto's Principle while focusing on The One **T**hing that's going to make the difference for you. So let's look at each of these parts of the formula in turn.

- **P**omodoro Technique:

At its simplest, the Pomodoro Technique involves working in 25-minute chunks with a 3-5 minute break between each chunk, followed by a longer 15–30-minute break after four sets. The overarching idea behind this technique is that frequent breaks help the brain to focus, which increases mental agility and efficiency. This is a powerful time management method developed by Francesco Cirillo in the 1980s as a result of the frustration he felt about how much time he wasted while he was studying. This led to him using a kitchen timer shaped like a tomato to boost his productivity. And that's how the Pomodoro Technique was born.

I love this because it gives us permission to push interruptions aside to focus on the task at hand. And the frequent breaks it involves gives us a chance to recharge so that we're refreshed and ready to go each time we sit down to work. What's more, there's no chance of burning out because we're only working in 25-minute bursts.

I think you'll be amazed at how much difference this part of the formula alone will make to the quality of your life, but wait until you read how simple the rest of the formula is.

- **G**ather:

The idea here is to gather all of the information you need for any given task in one place. I was actually stunned by the number of places I had to consolidate material from the first time I went through this process. So I thought I'd flag some of the places you're likely to find pieces of information that could be required for decision making and action taking in your own case. These include your calendar; email inbox and folders; task lists in software programs like MS Word and Note pad; text and voicemail messages on your mobile phone; personal Information managers (known as PIMs) like OneNote and Evernote; Customer Relationship Management systems (known as CRMs) like Salesforce; project management software like Basecamp and Slack; paperwork-on your desk; hand written notes in your purse; post-it-notes on the fridge; folders in filing cabinets; and last but not least, whatever you've got rattling around inside your head.

To be honest, it made me feel exhausted just writing these words down. I think I was a bit triggered because it reminded me of how discombobulated and stressful my life was when the information I needed to access was scattered all over the place.

- **P**areto Principle:

This is a tool that addresses the fact that there is an unequal relationship between inputs and outputs. The principle here is that 20% of the input we invest in completing a task is responsible for 80% of our results. The idea with the Pareto Principle is to ask yourself what are the 20% of actions that are driving 80% of the results you are getting in any particular area of your life, and then focus on those.

- **T**he One Thing:

Gary Keller takes the Pareto Principle to the next level in his book The One Thing. He focuses on the 20% of the 20% of the 20% until he gets down to ONE thing. Then he poses what he calls a 'Focusing Question'. That literally has the power to guide you directly to your core vision (or priority) in life. Being aware of your core vision makes it easier for you to make a decision about what things you are NOT going to do anymore.

So let me ask you – What's the One Thing you could do that will make everything else easier? Feel free to change the word 'easier' to one that works better for you. It could be:

- What's the One thing you could do that would relieve the pressure you're under?
- What's the One thing you could do that would repair your relationship with your partner?
- What's the One thing you could do to position yourself for a promotion?

F.A.S.T. Formula

I also use the F.A.S.T triaging formula to increase my productivity and (because of that) the quality time I get to spend with my family. What it does is help me move rapidly through actions, tasks, emails and projects by identifying what needs to happen with each item. It's ridiculously simple really. I literally organise everything that comes across my desk (including phone calls, emails, reading material, and the like) using the four dot points below.

- **F**ile it - There's no further action required, but it may be needed for reference later
- **A**ction it - It needs urgent action that will take less than two minutes
- **S**hift it/Schedule - Someone else can do it, or I can do it sometime in the future
- **T**rash it - No further action is required, and it won't be needed for future reference.

5. Business Savvy

There's no getting away from it (especially if you're like me and love your role as a doctor but feel like there's more to you than that, and wind up running a business on the side), it's important to recognise that we've been institutionalised to a certain extent, and we need to develop a whole new approach to operating if we want to become a successful entrepreneur. I'm using the words 'business savvy' here to encompass what I mean, because in order to run an efficient and successful practice, you need to know about things like sales and marketing. And you need to have the right systems and processes in place. What's more, if you employ staff, it's important to have the right team in place who've been through a robust onboarding strategy to empower them to perform at their best. These are the kinds of things that fall under the idea of 'business savvy'.

Sure, I know you might be paying someone to look after all of these things for you, but you still need to know the ins and outs of the business side of your business to ensure that everything is above board and sustainable.

What I know from first-hand experience is that it will serve you well to play the long game of entrepreneurship as you build your practice. From that perspective, it's worth checking in with yourself from time to time to make sure that you are continuously improving your skills in relation to business while you're developing your entrepreneurial mindset. And more specifically, it's important to be keeping an eye on whether you have the financial management skills to future-proof your business and ride out the storm in the event of cash flow or other problems emerging. And there's the question of having systems in place so that risk is minimised and operations run smoothly no matter what changes in the environment come to pass.

There's a reason the top entrepreneurial thinkers focus on growing their skills. And there's a reason why learning to become more entrepreneurial will help you weather any storm that may arise, and shift easily with the seasons of your business. If the global pandemic has taught us anything, it's to expect the unexpected and be ready to pivot as quickly and often as needed.

I feel like this is enough detail on the business side of transitioning into a heartfelt space for you to be taking on board right now. I'll be going much deeper on the question of mastering the art of entrepreneurship in my upcoming business book *The Heart-Centred Medical Entrepreneur* which is due for release in 2023.

———————————

Conclusion

What I want you to know is that I was where you may be heading not so long ago. I was a burnt-out pain specialist with dreams of finding a better way to keep doing the important work that I love, and I feel proud to share the points below that sum up my journey to developing my heart-centred business with you here. As I write this and reflect on what's happened since I starting to take the idea of becoming an entrepreneur seriously in December 2020, I can imagine people like you reading this book achieving similar outcomes:

- I am now known as the person behind the global brand I've established called The Heart-Centred Doctor.
- I'm a doctor with 15 years' experience and a well-known pain physician and expert in the fields of resilience and burnout.
- I run programs helping doctors transform their lives by moving from burnout to brilliance.
- I am a sought-after speaker and online educator.
- After a severe car accident in 2008, I was told I would never walk or practice medicine again. As a paraplegic my dreams were shattered. However, after digging deep and working on my mindset I managed to walk again after an intensive three-year recovery process.
- I have spoken at leading industry events including the Australasian New Zealand College of Anaesthesia and Faculty of Pain Medicine, where I raised the issue that

worries me most, which is the scourge of physician burnout, and how mindfulness and self-compassion can transform chronic pain.

- I have been featured in and written for Thrive Global, Yahoo Finance, International Business Times Singapore and Australian Business Journal.
- I have appeared in media regularly such as Sky News, Studio 10 and Ticker TV.
- I am co-authoring a book with Jack Canfield called Soul of Success Volume 3, which will be released in Spring 2022 in Los Angeles, California, USA.
- In addition to The Heart-Centred Medical Entrepreneur which will be released in 2023, my third book Radical Resilience will be released in early 2024.

The message for you here is that if I can achieve things like this, then so can you. If you would like a hand with your journey or more information about my Coaching and Leadership Programs, visit me at www.drolivialeeong.com.

References

Ashforth, B., 2012. *Role transitions in organizational life.* London: Routledge.

Brown, B., 2018. *Dare to Lead.* Penguin Random House UK.

Brown, B., 2016. *Daring Greatly: How the Courage to be Vulnerable Transforms the Way We Live, Love, Parent, and Lead.* London: Penguin Books Ltd.

Brown, B., 2010. *The Gifts of Imperfection: let go of who you think you're supposed to be and embrace who you are.* Hazelden Publishing.

Clarke-Fields., H., 2019. *Raising Good Humans, A Mindful Guide to Breaking the Cycle of Reactive Parenting and Raising Kind, Confident Kids.* Raincoast Books.

Cope, S.,2020. *Yoga and the Quest for the True Self.* Random House US.

Dweck, C., 2017. *Mindset: The New Psychology of Success.* Robinson.

Edmondson, A., 2008. *Teams that learn.* San Francisco, Calif.: Jossey-Bass Pfeiffer.

Germer, C. and Salzberg, S., 2009. *The mindful path to self-compassion.* New York: The Guilford Press.

Gladwell., M 2009 *Outliers.* London, Penguin Books.

Goleman, D., 2006. *Emotional intelligence.* New York, NY: Bantam Books.

Imms., A., 2019. *Burnout: Your first ten steps.* Australia.

Keller G., 2014. *The One Thing.* John Murray.

Neil M., 2013. *The Inside-Out Revolution.* Hay House UK Ltd.

Neff, K., n.d. *Self-compassion.*

Neff, K. and Germer, C., *The Mindful Self Compassion Workbook, A proven way to accept yourself, build inner strength and thrive*

Rosenberg B. M., 2015. *Nonviolent Communication.* Puddledancer Press.

Online Sources

Gottman., J article. The Greater Good Magazine. https://greatergood.berkeley.edu/article/item/john_gottman_on_trust_and_betrayal

Segel., D interview. The Therapist Uncensored Podcast. https://therapistuncensored.com/episodes/tu16-inside-the-mind-of-dr-dan-siegel-an-interview/

Heng., S., *Making Virtual Connections Meaningful in Our Near Normal.* https://simoneheng.com/making-virtual-connections-meaningful-in-our-new-normal/

Giurge M. Laura and Bohns K. Vanessa, *3 tips to avoid WFH Burnout*, Harvard Business Review. https://hbr.org/2020/04/3-tips-to-avoid-wfh-burnout

Prout S., *How to Manifest Anything You Want with the Law of Vibration*, 23 June 2015. How to Manifest Anything You Want with the Law of Vibration - Sarah Prout

Brene Brown On Connection (Article)
https://thekingandid.wordpress.com/2018/08/14/brene-brown-on-connection/

Australian Psychological Society. Stress.
https://www.psychology.org.au/for-the-public/Psychology-topics/Stress Accessed Sep 16, 2018.

Curtin M., *In an 8 hour day, the Average Worker is Productive for This Many Hours. It may make you feel better about leaving work early today.*
https://www.inc.com/melanie-curtin/in-an-8-hour-day-the-average-worker-is-productive-for-this-many-hours.html

www.ingramcontent.com/pod-product-compliance
Lightning Source LLC
Chambersburg PA
CBHW032146020426
42334CB00016B/1242